Praise for *Yoga for Cancer*

I am so thrilled to have found Vicky. My lymphoedema responds well to 'yoga for cancer', and I always feel buoyed by Vicky's compassion and caring. I do wonder if I might have escaped lymphoedema if I'd found Vicky during treatment; who knows! **Annemarie**

After just two classes with Vicky I started to feel back in my body. I connected with suppressed emotions in asanas Vicky taught – which was a welcome release after the months of tension and fear I had held on to. I began to unravel. If you are lucky enough to come across this remarkable and inspiring trauma-sensitive yoga therapist – wherever you are on your journey, embrace her and the process. She is a pure gift. Just when you may be giving up on the world. **Kate**

It turned out to be the best part of the complementary therapy I received. Not only did it distract my mind and strengthen my body through the lessons, but it equipped me with the mental tools to optimally deal with the treatment days, the scans, the hours spent in waiting rooms ahead of consultant appointments and the merits of mindfulness... there is a great deal of strength (physical and mental) that can be gained through yoga, all the more important during one of the most trying moments of one's life.

    The person who made this all happen was Vicky. She has such an experience with cancer patients that she is able to perfectly tailor her lessons to you – without asking too many probing questions. Because she just knows. I would actively encourage all men diagnosed with cancer to take up yoga as quickly as possible. **JR Robins**

I often have difficulty lying down (never mind beginning to move) because of the tumours in my ribs, sternum and spine. My mind naturally distracts me from the pain by thinking of other things. After an hour 'consciously breathing', I can feel the oxygen flowing in my body, I can expand my ribs without pain and be in the present moment (good and bad). I've now been able to stop all drugs for nausea and constipation through diet and yoga. **Tish**

I attended the 'yoga for cancer' class at Camden with Vicky Fox and it was wonderful. I'm hugely impressed that it is free, I love the setting, Vicky was kind and warm and understanding and the class itself was very well taught. I felt empowered and 'cared about' which is lovely after a gruelling year and a half of chemo, radiotherapy and surgeries. I came out of the class feeling relaxed, enthused and keen to return next week. Attending the class felt like a bit of the 'old me' was back and it has inspired me to do more yoga, mindfulness and breath work. This class and the very fact that someone thought to offer it means an awful lot to me. Thank you. **Triyoga student**

I came to realise a month or so ago (after much inner contemplation) that I had completely disconnected from my body – this actually served me well when undergoing chemo and painful surgeries etc – but definitely is not serving me well now – trying to get fit, tolerate the drugs I'm on and ultimately ward off a recurrence. I really haven't moved my body much at all the past 18 months or so – and I think I've been a bit scared to do so. Anyway, I was a bit nervous joining this morning but it was brilliant – a proper workout but I felt safe and supported at all times. I really feel like yoga is going to be the final missing piece in my recovery. I'm really looking forward already to the next class. Biggest thanks to you for offering this service. **Rachel**, online classes

Just wanted to say a huge thank you for everything this year; your positivity and absolutely fabulous classes have been a godsend to me. I thought it was medication and supplements that would help me on my healing journey, but actually it has been the mind–body connection that has been the most powerful, thank you. **Diane**, online classes

I wanted to say a special thank you for your advice on sleep problems. When I told you about my problems sleeping you explained a brilliant breathing technique to help me. Honestly, it has changed my life. I am now sleeping so much better. As soon as can't sleep I do the exact breathing method you showed me and I sleep. Thank you again. **Kim**

Yoga for Cancer
The A to Z of C

How yoga can reduce the side
effects of treatment for cancer

Vicky Fox

With Forewords by
Louise Malone and Deepa Morar

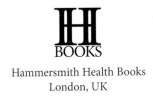

BOOKS
Hammersmith Health Books
London, UK

First published in 2022 by Hammersmith Health Books
– an imprint of Hammersmith Books Limited
4/4A Bloomsbury Square, London WC1A 2RP, UK
www.hammersmithbooks.co.uk

Disclaimer: This book is designed to provide helpful information on the subjects discussed. It is not meant to be used, nor should it be used, to diagnose or treat any medical condition. For diagnosis or treatment of any medical problem, consult your own physician or healthcare provider. The publisher and author are not responsible for any specific health or allergy needs that may require medical supervision and are not liable for any damages or negative consequences from any treatment, action, application or preparation, to any person reading or following the information in this book. References are provided for informational purposes only and do not constitute endorsement of any websites or other sources. Readers should be aware that the websites listed in this book may change. The information and references included are up to date at the time of writing but given that medical evidence progresses, it may not be up to date at the time of reading.

British Library Cataloguing in Publication Data:
A CIP record of this book is available from the British Library.

Print ISBN 978-1-78161-219-4
Ebook ISBN 978-1-78161-220-0

Commissioning editor: Georgina Bentliff
Typeset by: Bespoke Publishing Ltd
Cover design by: Madeline Meckiffe
Cover images: Shutterstock Merchgraphic (tree/figure) and bc21 (C-shape)
Index: Dr Laurence Errington
Production: Deborah Wehner of Moatvale Press Ltd
Printed and bound by: TJ Books, Padstow, Cornwall, UK

Contents

Foreword 1

Everyone needs a Vicky Fox in their life. As a healthcare practitioner and colleague of Vicky's, I am reassured by her knowledge and understanding of cancer, cancer treatments and the effect it has on the body and mind. Vicky also has a beautiful teaching manner, where she exudes warmth, empathy and compassion. The combination of both is unique and I truly believe the cancer world is a better place with her in it.

In my role as a Consultant Physiotherapist in Cancer Care, I know there is a wealth of evidence supporting exercise during cancer treatment. Not only does it help limit treatment-related side effects and keep people more functional during treatment, it can also reduce recurrence risk. But exercise does not mean going to the gym (I would say 95% of my patients have never stepped into one), it is about movement. It is about moving your body through breathwork, posture awareness, stretching, walking. It's about learning to be kind to your body, practising self-compassion, learning to let go and be comfortable in the way your body moves right now. All the beautiful things that can come from practising yoga.

I feel hugely privileged to work with Vicky and a question I love discussing with her and her students is: 'Is there a time when you can't practise yoga when you have cancer?' From my understanding, I believe the answer to be no. There will be times when other forms of exercise, activity and movement will not be possible. For example, after surgery, or when debilitated by treatment-related fatigue, or when the mind says go but the body says no, or the opposite; when the body says go but the mind says no. But yoga is always there. It is such a beautiful and powerful resource. From breathwork, mindfulness, stretching to strengthening, and guidance on lymphoedema management, I believe there is a time for yoga throughout all phases of cancer treatment.

I am so pleased that Vicky has published this book. I believe it will allow her to spread her wealth of knowledge and enable more to benefit from her skill and kindness. Whether you are someone undergoing treatment or perhaps a loved one looking for ways to support someone, this beautiful book will gently guide and empower you during and beyond this challenging time. I hope that you enjoy Vicky's words and benefit from her wisdom.

Louise Malone
Consultant Physiotherapist and Expert Practitioner in Oncology Care
www.louisemalone.com

Foreword 2

The approach to health and wellbeing is changing with the demand for non-pharmacological ways of managing symptoms ever increasing, particularly in the oncology field.

Many leading oncology hospitals around the world are now focusing on 'whole person care'. Integrative medicine embraces the biopsychosocial model addressing the body, mind, social and emotional aspects of healing.

Several evidenced-based modalities, like acupuncture, yoga, massage and mindfulness, are now woven alongside allopathic medicine, with overall better results to a more robust version of wellbeing.

It is remarkable that the ancient yoga has survived millennia, being testimony to its benefits, which are just as applicable and relevant in todays world. Yoga was originally designed as a preparation for meditation, with a focus to unite the body with the spirit. Yoga can be likened to a huge sun, whose rays can brighten so many aspects of our lives to bring clarity, healing and abundance.

The growing body of evidence is proving how yoga can benefit the musculoskeletal system by improving posture, flexibility, bone health, strength and cardiovascular health. There are numerous mental health benefits as well as to overall being, like improving sleep, which all contribute a greater overall quality of life.

Vicky Fox brings an immense effervescent energy to yoga coupled with her healing energy; she has assisted many people through their oncology journey. From first-hand knowledge, some have been so inspired to re-prioritise their lives and add this element of yoga into it that they have completed the yoga teacher training courses. Vicky provides a safe, caring space to heal.

It is one thing going through a journey of cancer and quite another one dealing with the side effects of active treatment. Here Vicky pulls together the numerous helpful threads of yoga to provide simple therapeutic ways to manage symptoms and optimise health.

The book is a simple, quick reference of A to Z, making it a user-friendly guide to anyone seeking to optimise their health and wellbeing.

Deepa Morar
Senior Physiotherapist, London Clinic

Acknowledgements

Thank you firstly to **all my students because you are my greatest teachers**. I am a permanent student and have learnt so much from teaching you all. Thank you for sharing your side effects, trusting in me and for giving me feedback on what worked and what didn't. I am so grateful.

I didn't get to write this book without all the trainings from senior teachers that shared with me their experiences and depth-of-knowledge. I couldn't have done this without you. Starting with Fred Busch who taught me how to be a yoga teacher, Laura Kupperman who trained me to teach Yoga For Survivors, Doug Keller for creating my passion for anatomy, Leslie Howard for detailed teachings and immense knowledge, Melina Meza for taking time to discuss spinal flexion with me - and for your wonderful classes, Rod Stryker for teaching me the energetics of sequencing – and Nicki Aylwin for sharing your meditation gems with me. Thank you to Golnaz Maleki for sharing your lymphoedema expertise, Zephyr Wildman for sharing your wisdom, Louise Malone (the best oncology physiotherapist), and Liliana Branco (the best specialist palliative care nurse).

Neil for always supporting and encouraging me (and taking the wonderful photographs) and Scarlet, Jack and Martha for grounding me. My mum Pat for patiently reading through the many versions of this so that I had something professional to send to Georgina Bentliff who agreed to publish this book and in doing so helps and supports people – we need more people like you in the world. And Peter and Sue for your constant positivity and support.

Special thanks to Jonathan Sattin for believing in me and giving me the opportunity to teach free classes in Triyoga's beautiful studios. Frankly none of this would have been possible without that opportunity and I am truly grateful for that.

Introduction

Since 2013 I have been teaching yoga to people diagnosed with cancer and have seen how yoga, which includes breathing, meditation, mantras and mudras, can have a huge benefit in reducing the side effects of treatment. I often tell people they don't need to feel good to come to a class, but they will feel better after a class.

We are all unique and individual, so a diagnosis of cancer is different for every person. No two cancers are alike. Every cancer treatment is tailor-made for that unique person, so what is true for one person may not be true for another.

How our body responds to treatment will be different from person to person. Treatment often damages healthy cells and tissue, and so side effects are common. However, some side effects are not commonly discussed, like constipation and premature menopause, and some seem common but are not, like losing your hair. Even if you are not having treatment, the one side effect of cancer common to all is anxiety, which can have a huge impact on your life.

According to Macmillan: 'There are now an estimated 2.5 million people living with cancer in the UK, a figure that is projected to rise to 4 million by 2030. Thanks to advances in treatment, people are now living longer with a cancer diagnosis than ever before. [...] This trend is expected to continue'[1]

More people are living longer with cancer and the side effects of cancer than ever before but, whilst the side effects are widely known, the support offered is often poor or even non-existent.[2]

So, the idea of this book is to look at some of the possible side effects, from Anxiety to ZZZZZ (sleep and insomnia), and see how we can use yoga to help with those symptoms. The book covers lymphoedema (fluid retention), osteoporosis (loss of bone strength), digestive dysfunction, fatigue, peripheral neuropathy (nerve problems in the extremities), loss of muscle mass and how we can quieten down our mind and take back some control.

However, just because there is a list of possible side effects of cancer and its treatment, it does not mean that you will experience all (or any) of them. Our mind is incredibly powerful, and research shows that what we *think* is what we experience, so just because these are *possible* side effects does not mean you will actually experience them. The scientific terms for the way the mind overrides reality in relation to illness and its treatment are 'placebo' and 'nocebo' effects:

- A placebo effect is where, for example, a patient is given a pill which they believe contains beneficial medicine (even though it does not), and they experience improvements in their health.
- The nocebo effect is the opposite; it is where, for example, a patient receives treatment which they believe will have a negative effect on their health (even though it is harmless), and this leads to a negative effect on their health.

Yoga practice can be supportive to you even if you aren't experiencing a particular side effect, as our bodies are designed to move – even though sometimes, over the course of cancer treatment, we may feel nervous about doing so. So, see each chapter in this book as empowering you to take back some control. There *are* things you can do to reduce the side effects of cancer treatment or make living with them more bearable.

What is yoga?

Firstly, it might be useful to explore what yoga actually is. To put it simply, I would describe yoga as breathing and 'breath-informed movement' to 'unstick' our tight bodies so that energy can thereby flow freely and with that create a settling of the mind. Breathing is an exceedingly powerful tool that we all have access to and that can very quickly change how we feel. Just a few minutes of conscious breathing can calm our mind and allow us to feel less reactive to our situation. However, I don't say any of this lightly because it can be very challenging to be still and to stay with your breathing when you are anxious, scared or fearful. This is where the movement comes in. I find it much easier to be able to sit and be still if I have moved my body first.

You might not have been able to move much during your cancer treatment, or you may have protected or guarded areas of your body and feel nervous of moving again.

The sequences in this book will address stretching into areas with a limited range of motion and poses that will build back strength so that daily activities, such as climbing stairs, should become easier. We need to move in a safe way so that we build back strength and flexibility slowly and mindfully and therefore safely. Yoga is a practice, not an achievement, and is something we can come back to again and again.

Can yoga help with cancer side effects?

The feedback I get from my in-person and online classes for people with a cancer diagnosis is very encouraging as you'll see from the examples quoted at the start of this book (pages i–ii).

Why exercise when you have cancer?

There are very good reasons for exercising. It can improve your quality of life and help you feel better. Regular exercise can reduce stress and give you more energy.

According to Cancer Research UK: 'Research has shown that there is strong evidence that certain ways of being active can help people with cancer:
- reduce anxiety
- improve depression
- reduce fatigue
- improve quality of life during and after cancer treatment
- prevent or improve lymphoedema (a type of swelling caused by treatment to lymph nodes)
- improve general physical functioning.'[3]

The US National Cancer Institute cites research that shows that exercise can help reduce breast, colorectal and prostate cancer mortality by 30–40%.[4]

A book that is well worth reading on the benefits of exercise for cancer patients is *Get Your Oomph Back: a guide to exercise after a cancer diagnosis*.[5] Carolyn Garritt is a cancer exercise expert and runs fitness classes through Maggie's Cancer Centres for anyone impacted by cancer.

Taking account of non-physical trauma and post-traumatic stress

Finally, it's important to acknowledge that some of my readers may have significant non-physical trauma through diagnosis and treatment. Traumatic events can lead to a severe anxiety disorder known as PTSD. In these situations, body scans and quiet non-moving mindfulness practices may be difficult and triggering, as can certain figures/asana. Trauma may mean you don't feel safe and therefore breathing or meditations with the eyes closed maybe triggering for you. If this is the case you might want to keep your eyes open and keep your gaze soft, or half-close your eyes so you are aware of the space around you. Breathing practices help to calm the parasympathetic side of the nervous system which is underactive in PTSD. When the parasympathetic side is stimulated, through breathing, we feel safer, less stressed and calmer and we release oxytocin (see the chapter on the Immune system, page 101). The physical practice of yoga can help bring us back into the present moment, into an awareness of 'now' and help you to find a relaxing pleasure in being in the present moment . Let your breath be your guide. If you are practising something that makes it harder for you to breathe, or you find you are holding your breath, then I would advise coming out of the physical pose you are in and back to a breathing practice that supports you. You might have a pleasant image or a visualisation that makes you feel safe and protected, which you might connect to when you feel anxious or overwhelmed. Grounding the body can help to make you feel that you are in a safe place. Feel the connection of your body to the ground and the earth beneath you, noticing which parts of your body actually make contact with the floor and sense how you are supported or held by the earth or the floor beneath you. You might find using an affirmation such as 'I am loved', 'I am safe' or 'I am protected', or other supportive words that make you feel safe, will help and bring you into the 'now'.

Integrative Medicine Doctor, Scientist and Educator, Dr Nina Fuller-Shavel has shared this important advice:

'If during any practice or outside of it, there are intrusive thoughts or memories related to diagnosis, persistent signs of nervous system dysregulation (particularly if related to specific triggers) or distressing feelings arising that the person does not feel able to manage, they should speak to their GP, oncology team or integrative doctor to be evaluated more formally for PTSD and to get support. There is a possibility of trauma resulting from both diagnosis and treatment and therefore it may be necessary to seek help. Unfortunately, some studies show that one-third of patients with breast cancer who were initially diagnosed had persistent or worsening PTSD four years later, potentially because of a lack of prompt and appropriate intervention, which we want to avoid. In my mind, awareness of cancer-related PTSD with prompt diagnosis and appropriate treatment is really important, as well as broader trauma response awareness even if full PTSD criteria are not fulfilled.'

How to use this book

There is a paradox that the treatment for cancer is actually what makes you feel worse, and it is often the side effects of treatment that are challenging to live with and not the cancer itself. This book addresses those side effects and how yoga can support or ease the symptoms.

This is a book that you don't have to read from cover to cover but can dip in and out of at will to access information about a specific side effect or symptom that is relevant to you in that moment. There are also related videos for each letter of the alphabet on vickyfox-yoga.com.

This book looks at breathing exercises (**pranayama**), physical postures (**asana**), hand gestures (**mudras**), sounds (**mantras**) and meditation that can support, ease and make life more comfortable. You don't need to feel well to practise the sequences, but you will feel better for taking the time for yourself to breathe and move. You can practise from six weeks post-surgery, as long as all surgical incisions have healed, and whilst you are going through treatment. You will find that certain exercises and poses are repeated through the book as they are helpful with a range of symptoms.

If you have a PICC (peripherally inserted central catheter) there are no specific guidelines for doing yoga, but this book focuses on moving in a safe and pain-free way. I have taught hundreds of people with PICC lines and they have found benefit in keeping their arm moving and enjoyed being in class reaping the other benefits of yoga. You might feel nervous moving your arm, but you will be able to find a pain-free range of movements that work for you. We don't do big weight-bearing poses on the arms in yoga for cancer as this is contraindicated.

If you have a port-a-cath, this is sealed under the skin, so if all incisions have healed, then it is safe to practise yoga with a port.

The chapter on 'Colostomy, ostomy, ileostomy and yoga with a stoma' (page 59) will help if you are nervous of moving with a stoma. You can feel reassured that the practices described in that chapter are designed to release tension and build strength in a safe way.

I should also say that the poses in this book are just a guide. You are actually your best teacher as you are the only person who knows what it feels like to be in your body. This may change from day to day and moment to moment. Yoga is an individual practice. Take time to notice how you feel. Observe how you feel without judging or labelling sensations as 'good' or 'bad'. When we start to quieten our mind and stop analysing and judging we can notice how we truly feel in that present moment.

Your body talks to you through subtle sensations, so observe these sensations and notice how it feels. If you find you can no longer breathe smoothly, or something feels uncomfortable or painful, then you need to ease out of a pose a bit or completely. You can use this book to do what feels right for you on each individual day. Some days you may be full of energy and looking for something to help you build strength and improve your flexibility. On other days, you may feel exhausted or depleted of energy and need a practice that is more restorative. You might follow a complete sequence or just pick some poses from the sequence to fit your need or the time you have to practise.

Kindness

In yoga philosophy there are guidelines on how to live a meaningful and purposeful life. They are known as the 'eight limbs of yoga'.[1] The very first limb of yoga is **ahimsa**. Ahimsa means non-harming or non-violence – that is, non-harming in the way we treat others and ourselves. We can think of this as physical in terms of not pushing into pain, but also in the way we speak to ourselves. How often are we mean to ourselves or speak to ourselves in a way that we would never dream of addressing another person? So, becoming more aware of how we are speaking to ourselves, starting to be aware of our habits to see if we are practising ahimsa in our lives, and realising that being kind *is* 'doing yoga'. Ahimsa is not just the absence of violence, but is the presence of love. Be kind to yourself always.

If you experience pain, it is important that you recognise that and back off. You may have intense or 'pulling' sensations when working with scar tissue or areas you have guarded, but it should not feel like pain. Let your breathing guide you and if you are holding your breath, waiting for a movement or pose to be over, then you need to ease out of it. The shape of your breathing is more important than the shape of your pose, so if you can't breathe fully or your breathing becomes erratic, change the shape of the pose so you can breathe fully and evenly.

I think the power of kindness is underrated; kindness also means being non-judgemental and inclusive and is one of the most powerful qualities we can have as a human being. Kindness can be seen as being wimpy or weak, but knowing when you need to back off and when you need to take it easy is incredibly important when trying to repair, nourish and nurture ourselves. It is easy to be judgemental and critical when we can't do things we previously could do easily. However, we are not required to accept every thought that comes into our mind and, when we begin to observe our thoughts, we can start to see which of them might not be true, kind or generally not really serve any purpose. By reading this book you have become a co-crafter of your wellbeing. You are part of your treatment plan and are taking control.

Responding to change

Change is an integral part of life, and it can feel like a threat, but coming to terms with, and learning to accept, change is part of the practice of yoga. We can't change what life throws at us, but we can change how we respond to it. Responding with frustration or kindness to our changing situation can make life harder or easier and we can choose which we would prefer. Jon Kabat-Zin in *Full Catastrophe Living* describes healing as 'coming to terms with things as they are'.[2] Yoga helps us to be more present and in the moment with whatever that moment brings and when we are fully in this moment then we have more energy for living. We use up a lot of energy when we are wishing we are somewhere else, doing something else or wishing something was different.

You can ask yourself: 'Is your current situation something that you can change?' If the answer is 'yes', then do you have the energy to try to change the situation and is it worth it? If the answer is 'no' then can you approach your situation in a kind way, starting to accept that this is something that can't be changed even if you would desperately like to. Accepting does not mean that we like the way things are but that we become willing to see things *as* they are. This can give you a sense of being in control which can be exceedingly empowering if you currently feel that life is out of your control.

Connection

Furthermore, when we are kind, we generally feel better about ourselves, something we will explore further in the chapter on the 'Immune system and infections' (page 101). Being kind to others and to ourselves connects us because being compassionate to ourselves and others helps us to realise that we are not so different to each other. Part of being human is the desire to avoid suffering and to feel contented with what we have in life.

When we feel we are all connected and all part of a bigger picture we also feel less isolated or lonely and this can lead to increased social bonds. Studies have shown that we all thrive better in a community. For example, one study found that women with metastatic breast cancer who had a weekly support group lived on average twice as long as the group of women who didn't have a support group.[3] It has not been possible to replicate the Spiegel *et al.* study, but there are many other studies looking at how those who are supported live longer than those who don't. For example, Fawzy *et al* found that a group of patients who didn't receive support were twice as likely to have a recurrence of cancer as those who received support.[4] Other studies show that not only do people live longer when they have social connections, but they also have lower cancer rates.[5, 6, 7]

When we are no longer struggling to survive or feeling that we are constantly battling or fighting, we may just start to feel the sense of contentment or peace that is always within us. Our immune system and our ability to defend ourselves is less effective when we are in conflict, and finding some connection to ourselves, and then maybe others, can help us feel like we belong. With that sense of belonging, we can be more comfortable in our own bodies, being who we truly are and feeling at peace within our own skin.

Repairing on many levels

Healing is a process of becoming whole, so when looking at yoga as a way of healing or repairing it is worth noting that the yoga tradition views the body as multi-layered and multi-dimensional; these layers are known as the **koshas**. We are magnificent beings that mostly connect to our body on its most physical and gross level. This is the layer of body that we are aware of changing, especially with a cancer diagnosis. Some of these physical changes are permanent and some are temporary, some are obvious, and some are hidden. The asana, or physical practices, will help us move the physical body or **annamaya kosha**.

To heal though (and when I speak of healing, I mean creating this sense of whole-ness or a sense of balance in the body), we can start to look at the other layers of the body and repair on many levels and not just on a physical level. All the layers are linked so you can't affect one layer without it influencing another.

The breath or energetic body known as the **pranayama kosha** is a more subtle layer and may be harder to be aware of. However, you may have experienced the feeling of walking into a room where there has been an argument and being able to sense that the energy of the room feels negative, and there's that expression that you could 'cut the atmosphere with a knife'. Energy is everywhere around us and within us, moving and vibrating in waves and particle forms. We get energy from food and water and from people and nature, but we also get our energy from our breath. The vital energy or life force that flows through the body is known in the yoga tradition as **prana**.

Yoga can give you more opportunity to stop and observe this energetic layer of the body. Sometimes this may be as obvious as noticing whether you are full of energy or depleted of energy. It might also be noticing areas of your body that feel more awake or alive, where the life force or prana is flowing freely. Or noticing where you feel your breath moving in your body and if your breath is getting stuck anywhere. Where we guide our awareness, breath and energy can follow so we can breathe into areas that feel stuck or tight.

At the beginning of your yoga practice, you can start by stopping. Stopping to notice not how you 'think' you might feel but how you actually feel. Being diagnosed with cancer literally takes your breath away and changing how you breathe has an effect on your physical body. Our breath is automatic but also voluntary and we can change how we breathe to start to change how we feel, because our breath is the quickest way to impact our nervous system. So, some of the practices in this book look at exercises that focus on breathing or that focus on subtle movements of energy through hand gestures (mudras) that help to redirect or concentrate energy in one location.

Energy is distributed to nourish our muscles, organs and cells through a complex system of energy channels known in yoga as **nadis**. Our physical body depends on energy (or prana) for its wellbeing as energy fuels the nervous and circulatory systems. When our energy is depleted, we can sometimes describe the feeling as being 'burnt out' and this will have a knock-on effect on our body and mind.

Our mind includes our thoughts, judgements, concepts, patterns and ways of thinking and it is in our mind that we absorb and process all our experiences. It is here in our mental body, or **manomaya kosha**, that we try to make sense of it all. Our mind swings from the past to the future, spending very little time in the present moment. But the present moment is the only place that you *can* be in. We suffer when we focus on what happened in the past and rehash things that have been and gone. We also suffer when our mind is in the future worrying about things that might happen but might never. I once read that worrying was projecting fearfully into an imaginary future which we can't cope with because it doesn't exist. We don't have a crystal ball so who knows what the future might bring.

Patanjali's Yoga Sutras[1] are 195 short teachings or threads called **sutras** concerned with the nature of the mind and the way the mind works. These texts, although written around 200 BCE–400 AD, look at the effects on our lives when our minds are agitated, and are probably even more relevant now than when they were written. In sutra 1.2, Patanjali defines yoga as the 'calming control of the repetitive disturbances of the mind': Yogas-citta-vrtti-nirodhah.

When we are not being disturbed by our mind, we might start to experience a sense of peace that is always within us, a glimpse of our true nature. This has been confirmed by scientific studies, which have shown that women with breast cancer who participated in a six-week course of yoga found significant improvements in anxiety, depression and perceived stress.[8]

When we start to move our physical body (annamaya kosha), get better connected to our breath (pranamaya kosha) and can observe our thoughts (manomaya kosha) without judgement, then we can become more in tune and start to access our intuitive or wisdom body, **vijnyanamaya kosha**. When we judge others, this can create a sense of separation rather than a sense of cohesiveness, and I think this makes us feel more isolated or lonely because it highlights how different we are from others rather than reminding us that, in reality, we are all the same with the same desires to be healthy and free from pain and suffering. Judgements can also make us less open to new things or close off our hearts, which from an energetic perspective can affect the flow of energy through the body.

You might even make judgements reading this book. I wonder if you can read it with an open heart and a beginner's mind? See if you can be open to new things without labelling them as 'a bit far out' or 'not my cup of tea'. Maybe through some of the practices in this book you can become more connected to your feelings and sensations, and to your inner sense of the world.

The western world often overlooks the profound intelligence in the body that we sometimes feel in the physical and emotional centre of our body, our gut. A 'gut feeling' is a thought or sensation about something that logic can't explain. We speak of our gut when describing someone with courage or strength as 'having guts'. We also might have experienced that sinking feeling in our tummies when something goes wrong, or we do not experience the outcome we have wished for.

Our intellect might try to talk us out of our gut feelings as our mind applies logic to those feelings, but if you quieten your mind through meditation, breathing and yoga you might just start to hear the quiet inner voice of intuition.

The kosha model is based on interconnectedness, which means that our thoughts affect our energy which in turn affects our physical body. There is no separation. When we feel disconnected this does not help our wellbeing and, through yoga, we can start to cultivate a connection to our true nature. Our true nature is the sense of self we were born with, the part of us that gets buried in our socially-created self or our self that has been diagnosed with cancer. You might notice that, at the end of a yoga practice, you can sometimes get a glimpse of this true nature and sometimes that feels calm or peaceful as you connect to your **anandamaya kosha** or bliss body.

Patanjali says that deep within each one of us is our true self and that the true self is luminous, clear and bright.[1] When our mind is agitated it obscures that light and muddies it, but if we can settle our mind and find an inner calmness, then we can start to be aware of this inner light or true nature. When we feel more serene or content, then we might be more comfortable with change because within us our true self is constant and inherently peaceful and calm. Outside of us, things are constantly in flux and change is a natural part of life, but if our inside stays calm then we might just learn to be okay with the perfectly imperfect world around us? Although things are not going to be the same again *that* is okay.

You might have felt like you wanted to run away from your body, especially with it changing physically, but this multi-dimensional approach can actually give you the opportunity to connect more strongly to this wonderful, magnificent, multi-layered but challenging body that you live in. Then you might feel that connection to something else, to people who empower us, to people who inspire us, to people who support us. Connect to something greater, find a purpose and, through this experience, the union of yoga; then we can start to repair on these many levels.

Mudras

Some of the yoga practices are subtle and work on the energetic or breath body, like the mudras or hand gestures included in some chapters. I have included these as they can be done by anyone, at anytime and anywhere. Even if you have days in hospital or are too fatigued to move, then you can practise a hand gesture or mudra to explore the effects. Mudra translates as 'to seal' or 'gestures', and in this book we will be focusing on the hands to guide energy, focusing it in certain areas or stop it being dissipated.

Have you ever put your fingers together to touch when you are trying to remember something? We cross our fingers when we want to wish someone good luck, we clap our hands to show appreciation and some hand gestures may be considered offensive. The placement of our hands can be really powerful and, if I feel disconnected or upset, I will often place my hands on my heart to give me a sense of calm and grounding. So maybe you already naturally do something with your hands or maybe you will find a mudra in this book that works for you.

There is no scientific evidence to support mudras, but we have a strong neural connection between our hands and our brain, and our fingers give our brain information all the time. Through the nerves and our connective tissue our hands tell us if a surface is hot or cold, rough or smooth. So, in reverse, can we send messages of love or repair from our brain to our hands? It is definitely worth exploring, isn't it? In reflexology parts of the fingers and hands are seen as connected to parts of the body. In Traditional Chinese Medicine, stimulating the meridian lines in the fingers and hands can relieve a symptom somewhere else in the body. In Ayurveda yoga, the fingers represent the elements. The thumb is fire, the index finger air, the middle finger ether, the ring finger earth and the little finger water. From a yogic perspective, they help to direct energy to areas of the body that might need it or help concentrate energy or prana in a certain area.

Before practising with mudras, it is often good to sit and just observe your breathing. Notice what your breath feels like. Notice where it is more dominant. Front of body? Sides of body? Back of body? Does your breath get stuck anywhere? Can you breathe down into your belly? Is it easier to breathe down one side of your body than the other?

Then, when you do focus on your hands, you will be able to gauge if anything changes with your breathing or to notice what has changed. Start by sensing where your fingers touch. Pay attention to your breathing, again noticing if it is more challenging to breathe with the mudra. If it *is* more challenging, then I would release that mudra and try a different one.

Sometimes you can also direct your breath into your hands or a particular area of your body. Energy follows awareness. Try it yourself. Close your eyes and bring your awareness to your right hand. Notice what changes. Does it become warmer? Are you aware of movement of energy? Do you feel swirling sensations in your palm or does your palm feel more zingy or energised?

Guidelines for working with mudras

- Start slowly. Make sure the mudra feels okay with a few breaths and then build up to a practice of 1 minute then maybe, over time, to 5 minutes.
- Go with your intuition. You might observe that your hands naturally find a mudra when you come to sit in meditation and some mudras might be preferable to others.
- Mudras should feel pleasant and/or supportive. Subtle is best.
- Try working with one mudra for a period of time, perhaps a few weeks; it can take a while to become aware of any subtle differences.

Mantras and sound to help to repair

Our English language has been influenced by many different cultures all competing with each other – for example, our word for 'pen' could very easily have been the French word 'stilo' but instead is from the Latin for a 'feather'. Sanskrit words were said to have been given to enlightened people like seers or rishis in their dreams and meditations, and the syllables are said to be embedded with energy, which is why chanting a mantra can be so powerful. However, if you find that repeating Sanskrit words does not resonate with you and you have an affirmation, or two positive English words that sit better with you, then you could try repeating these whilst you breathe. You might mentally say 'healthy' as you breathe in and 'strong' as you breathe out, or 'calm' as you inhale and 'centred' as you exhale.

We often work in class with the mantra **so ham** (pronounced 'so hum'). This mantra mimics the sound of the breath and can be a focus for your mind so that you get a break from your thoughts, allowing your mind and body to start to calm. 'So ham' is Sanskrit and translates as 'I am that'. '*So*' means 'I am' and '*ham*' means 'that'. This is referring to 'that' which is living and existing through us all. Hear the whisper of 'so' as you breathe in. Hear the whisper of the sound 'hum' as you breathe out. In an article for *Yoga International*, Rolf Sovik says of *so hum* that 'all that is needed is a genuine willingness to let the sound become the relaxed focus of attention. Then the coordination of breath and sound can have its natural effect on the mind and personality'.[9]

So ham helps us to remember that we are all part of something bigger and that we are all connected, and this connection can help us feel less isolated or lonely, especially at night-time when this feeling can be especially intense.

Exploring sound and the vibrations that it makes

Find a comfortable seated position with your spine long and weight equal in your sitting bones. Bring your right hand to your throat and rest your left hand on top of your right hand. Take a breath in and as you exhale hum 'mmmmmmmmmmmmmm'. Observe what you feel under your hands and through your hands. Can you feel the vibration that the sound creates?

Now try some different sounds, such as vowel sounds a, e, i, o and u. Do these sounds create different vibrations and where do you feel these sounds resonate in your body?

Sound travels in wave form. Sound waves can travel through water, and we are around 60% water. The vibrations that the sound waves create can ripple down through our body and start to massage our internal organs with the pulsations of the waves.

It might also explain why some people enjoy singing and chanting, because the sounds made when we sing or chant come from contracting our vocal cords and creating a resistance in our throat, which creates sound waves; these stimulate the vagus nerve (see page 49), which in turn soothes the parasympathetic nervous system (see page 49) and makes us feel good. Also, when we sing, we slow down the exhale; a longer exhale is more calming to the nervous system.

The following **bija** or seed mantras (one-syllable mantras) come from the *Vedas*, a vast collection of ancient philosophical teachings from India. These single syllables are mantras that, according to yoga tradition, are sounds that carry different energies or 'prana'. These sounds might bring some balance to areas that are out of balance or need some love or tender loving care. So, if there is an area of your body you want to direct energy or vibration into, then you could try the sound that the ancient yogis placed on that area of the energetic body. You can chant these sounds and see if any of the sounds resonate in your body. They can be done seated or lying down or whilst moving in and out of yoga poses.

Lam (pronounced 'lum'). Lam brings awareness to the grounding of your legs or sitting bones if you are seated, or to your feet if you are standing. Feel the earth beneath you and direct the sound down to the base of your pelvis and feel how the ground beneath you holds and supports you.

Vam (pronounced 'vum'). Vam brings awareness down to your lower belly. You could place a hand above your pubic bone and sense the vibrations of 'vam' reverberate down your body to your pelvis. You could move your pelvis forward and back in a small rocking motion to direct the sound down into your lower belly.

Ram (pronounced 'rum'). Ram brings awareness down into the abdomen and lower back, it visualises the sound waves massaging down into the digestive system and senses the vibrations of the sound stimulating the organs of the belly.

Yam (pronounced 'yum'). Yam brings awareness to the heart, lungs and thoracic spine. Place a hand on your heart and feel the sound vibrate down into your chest. Sense the organs of your chest all being massaged by the sound 'yam'. Can you feel the sound in the back of your body as well as the front? You can place a hand at the back of your heart to sense the movement of your breath into the space in between your shoulder blades.

Ham (pronounced 'ham'). Ham brings awareness to the throat; place a hand on your throat to sense the vibrations there when you chant 'ham'. Sense your throat as the centre of communication and your ability to speak and to fully express your thoughts and feelings. So, sense sending energy into this area to be able to find your voice and be able to communicate what you want to with ease.

Om. Bring your awareness to the roof of your mouth and the point between your eyebrows and where these two points might meet in your head. As you chant 'om', sense the sound vibrating here and sense this area as helping you to have clear thinking and perception; focusing here may help you be more intuitive.

Where to start

Props and other tips

I find it is really helpful to create a space to practise that is personal to you and can feel a little bit like a mini sanctuary, putting your phone on silent and moving away from the distractions of computers or work so that you signal to yourself that this is 'My time' – time that you are taking out of your day to put yourself first. Is there a good time of day when you know you are less likely to be disturbed? Can you let people around you know that you are taking time out for 'you'?

A yoga mat can be a good investment and the simple act of rolling out your mat starts to put you into the headspace and frame of mind that you are now taking control and time to nurture and nourish youself. To create clear pictures, the photographs in this book don't actually show a yoga mat but I highly recommend having something that makes it more comfortable and padded to lie down onto and also might stop you sliding when you are in standing poses. Some mats have a stickiness to them that allows your feet to grip and not slip.

We use props in yoga to elevate the floor when it doesn't quite meet us or to lengthen our arms when they are just not long enough to reach something. Props are really useful to make poses accessible to all of us and this is especially important when we might need to modify poses due to scar tissue, tight areas or other issues, like lymphoedema, that can limit our range of movement. Throughout lockdown we modified using tin cans or dictionaries instead of blocks, and scarves or belts instead of yoga straps. So, you can be creative in how you modify things. However, if you find that yoga is helpful to you, then it might be worth investing in a couple of yoga bricks (brick-sized yoga blocks), a strap and a bolster. Straps can come in a variety of lengths and it is worth buying a long strap for some of the restorative poses as this might be more useful to you than a shorter strap. Bolsters are really useful in restorative poses and great for lying over to open up the chest and release tension. You can create a bolster yourself by rolling a pillow lengthways in a towel or blanket. If you are looking to purchase yoga equipment, then Yogamatters.com has a great selection of yoga props.

A simple daily sequence

The following sequence is great for warming up the body before adding on any further poses, for aiding digestion and for getting the whole body moving.

The opening sequence brings movement into your arms, legs and core and allows you to start to connect your breathing with movement. In addition, because it is done supine (lying down) it can be done on days when you are feeling fatigued or low in energy. As the movements are with the breath, you can experience the union of breath and movement, and the repetitions allow us to warm up and find more space or more release with each repetition. Moving with our breath is called **vinyasa yoga**, which also translates as 'to place in a special way'. So, see if you can link your breath with the movement. Where there are repetitions of poses, you can repeat these as often as you want or as many times as you have time for. To make it more challenging you can increase the number of repetitions or hold the poses for longer, or to make it easier, have fewer repetitions and shorter holds. However, it is **quality not quantity** that matters here – quality of movement and of breath.

Opening sequence

- Start on your back in constructive rest pose: knees bent, feet flat on the floor in line with your hip sockets.
- Place a support under your head. Feel the weight of your head, ribs and pelvis. Notice the space between your lower back and the floor and your neck and the floor. There might not actually be space between your lower back and the floor, but your lower back should not be flattened or squashed.
- Also notice if the curve in your neck is exaggerated (see Figures 1 and 2); if

it is, this is incorrect, and you may need to adjust the support under your head in order to bring your neck into a neutral position (see Figure 3).

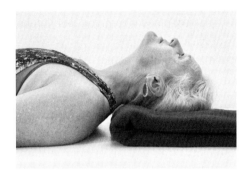

Figure 1: Head tipped too far back – incorrect

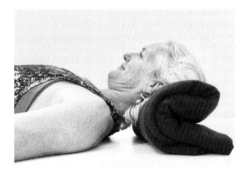

Figure 2: Head tipped too far forward – incorrect

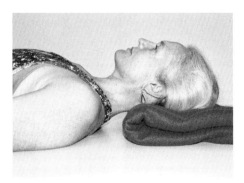

Figure 3: Head supported in a neutral position – correct

- Another adjustment to try if this doesn't feel very restful is to move your knees in towards each other. You could even put a prop between your knees to rest them on.
- Then move your feet either a little wider apart or a little closer together and see if there is a perfect place where you feel you have created a space between your lower back and the floor.
- Then lie in this position and just breathe.

Take time to notice what you are bringing to your practice. Observe your body and the different layers, as described on page 8. What does it feel like in your physical body today? What are your levels of energy? What is your prevailing mood? What is the quality of your thoughts? Can you bring your awareness to your breath and breathe in fully and out fully? Observe where in your body you feel breath. Is it easier to breathe in some areas of your body than others? Can you guide your breath to the areas that feel stuck?

This is a fabulously simple pose that allows your body to relax and gravity to draw you down into the floor. It helps to release your hip flexor muscle, the psoas, which is one of your fight or flight muscles that can get tight from stress but also from spending time seated.

Arm exercises

Next, start making 'snow angels' with your arms.
- Slide your arms back towards your ears as you **inhale** and then back down to your sides as you **exhale**.
- Just explore the range of motion in your shoulders. Keep the range of motion pain free, although you might meet intensity. Repeat 3–4 more times, moving with your breath (see Figures 4 and 5).

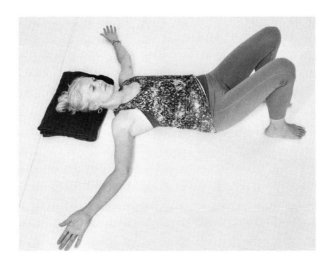

Figure 4: Sliding arms up as you inhale

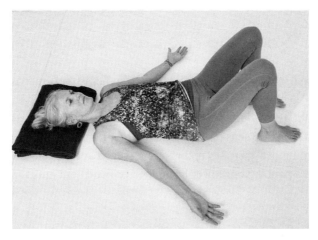

Figure 5: Sliding arms down as you exhale

Arm exercise with vinyasa

- Next, stretch your arms up to the ceiling and interlace your fingers so if you have an arm with a limited range of motion it can be supported by a stronger arm (see Figure 6).

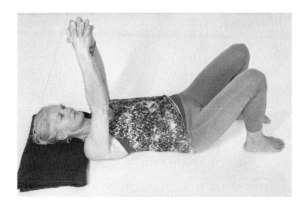

Figure 6: Arm stretch with interlaced fingers

- **Inhale** and stretch your arms back towards your ears. I emphasise the word 'towards' as they may not go that far but you are working in that direction and should be moving in a pain-free way. It can feel intense, and you might experience pulling sensations but no pain. You might feel comfortable straightening out your legs at this point, so you get a whole-body stretch. If this causes pain in your lower back, then re-bend your knees (see Figure 7).

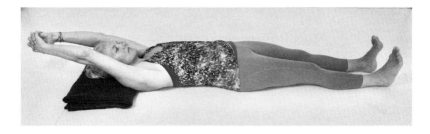

Figure 7: Whole-body stretch as you inhale

- Then, as you **exhale**, hug your right knee in towards you, trying not to curl your pelvis off the floor as you move your right leg (see Figure 8).

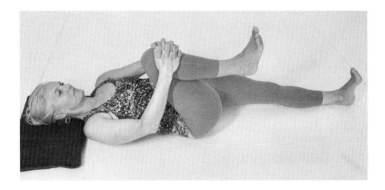

Figure 8: Hugging right knee in as you exhale

- Repeat this vinyasa for a few more rounds of breath.

Knees and toes

- Then, next time you **exhale**, hug your right knee in and keep it there; circle your ankle in one direction 4–5 times and then in the other 4–5 times so you lubricate your ankle joints.
- Then, as you **inhale**, extend your leg and point your toes (see Figure 9); as you **exhale** re-bend your knee and flex your foot (see Figure 10).

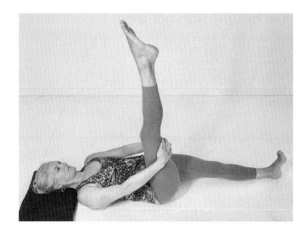

Figure 9: Extending leg and pointing toes as you inhale

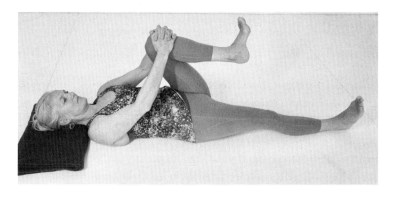

Figure 10: Re-bending knee and flexing foot as you exhale

- If this causes you any discomfort in your lower back, bend your left knee and plant your foot on the floor. Easing into your hamstrings, repeat this movement 4–5 times.

Hamstrings

Hamstrings get tight when we are spending time seated and they become shortened and don't get stretched so you might find that yours are tight. This exercise feels like you are flossing your muscles and the neural pathways that run through them.

- Bend your left knee and cross your right ankle over your left thigh or, if that is not comfortable, then your right heel on top of your left knee.
- Flex your feet (see Figure 11).

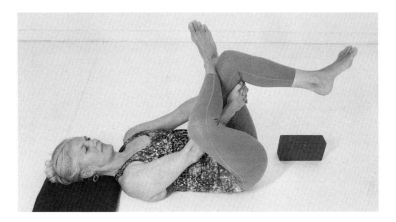

Figure 11: Figure-of-four stretch for glutes

- You could stay in this position or firm your belly and elevate your left foot onto a yoga block or draw your left knee in towards you. If this causes any strain to your chest or arms you can use a strap to reach through to hold your leg, or bring your left foot back to the floor and put a yoga block underneath it.
- Stay in this position for 5–8 breaths.
- Release and stretch back out and repeat on the other side, hugging your left knee in and circling your ankle.

Thigh muscles

- Bring your feet back to the floor or mat and, keeping your knees bent, widen your feet to the edges of the mat.
- **Exhale** and take your knees over to the left. **Inhale** and breathe into the right side of your chest (see Figure 12).
- **Exhale** and bring your knees back to face the ceiling and then over to the right. **Inhale** and breathe into the left side of your chest, softening your left shoulder (see Figure 13).

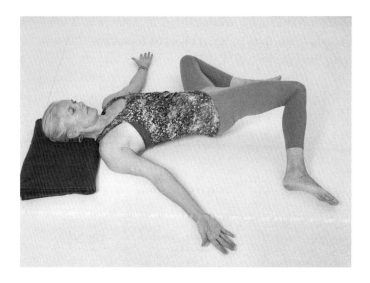

Figure 12: Taking knees over to the left as you exhale and breathing into right side of chest as you inhale

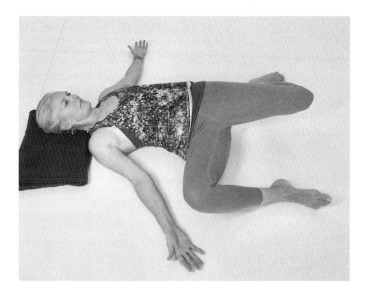

Figure 13: Taking knees over to the right as you exhale and breathing into left side of chest as you inhale

- Continue this windscreen-wiper movement with your legs 3–4 more times on each side, moving to the other side on your exhale.
- Then take your knees over to the left and pause here.
- Press your right knee away from your right hip to get a stretch along the quadricep (thigh muscle) and hip flexors (top of thigh/groin). If you feel it in your lower back, you can try putting your hands on your rib cage and drawing your ribs in, so they don't stick out into your clothing. You could also place a block or cushion under your left leg to elevate the floor. You could also draw your tailbone into your body and your pubic bone towards your belly button to lightly engage your core and protect your lower back.
- Stay in this position for 8 breaths and then repeat on the other side.
- Finally, hug your knees into your chest (see Figure 14) and circle your knees in one direction and then the other, 3–4 times each. If you want, you can take your hands away from your knees and, keeping the shape of your spine, circle your knees without your hands. Your tummy muscles will work to stop your back from arching away from the floor and keep your spine neutral. If this feels like too much, then bring your hands back to your knees.

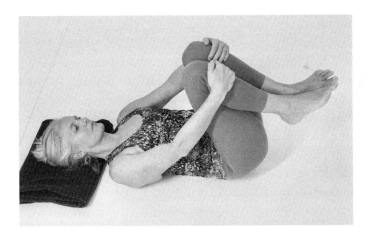

Figure 14: Hugging knees to chest

To finish: savasana

Bring your feet back down to the mat and, if comfortable, slide out your legs and take about 5 minutes just to absorb your short practice (see Figure 15). Notice if anything has changed and take a moment to let go physically.

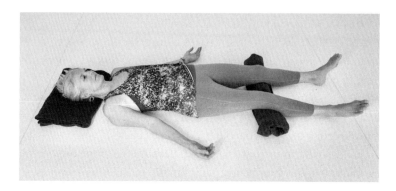

Figure 15: Relax (savasana)

Allow your body to be heavy and sink down into the ground, your mat or bed. Let go of your breath so you are no longer consciously shaping it, just feeling your body being breathed. Can you allow your mind to settle with the breath? Let go of anything that doesn't serve you any purpose – attachments you have made during your sequence; the things you 'liked' and 'disliked' or felt you 'did well' or weren't so 'good at'. Let them go for a few minutes and just take time being and not doing.

This pose is called **savasana** and is one of the most important poses we do in our yoga practice; it gives us a chance to absorb everything we have done and to observe how we feel in this moment. Sometimes in savasana we get a glimpse of our true nature – the nature we were born with. So, take a few minutes here, if you can, to let go, absorb and notice. To be a human being, not a human doing, and to get the huge benefits of doing nothing.

Savasana can sometimes be the hardest pose to be in as we are not distracted by any movement and, when we are still, we can suddenly be aware of how noisy our mind is. If you find that it is really hard to be fully conscious, you could try either coming back to following your breath or to using the mantra *'so ham'* (pronounced 'so hum' – see page 13). *'So ham'* can help us to gather and focus our energy on the repetition of sound. As you **inhale**, hear the sound *'so'* on your breath. As you **exhale** hear the sound *'ham'* as you breathe out. Continue hearing the sound *'so ham'* on your breath as you breathe in and out. As your mind wanders, gently bring it back to the mantra.

You can include *so ham* in any of the practices in this book. Some students in my classes have found this mantra useful when they have been waiting for results or having scans or chemo. Anytime you find your mind is really busy, see if giving it another focus helps to calm it. If you feel any resistance to *so ham*, then you could try instead mentally saying 'let' as you breathe in and 'go' as you breathe out: 'let – go'. See if following 'let' on inhale and 'go' on exhale helps you to release and let go.

When you are ready to come out of the daily sequence, roll to the side that is most comfortable for you. This may mean keeping a stronger arm on top to help press into the floor. Let your head be the last thing to come up (see Figure 16).

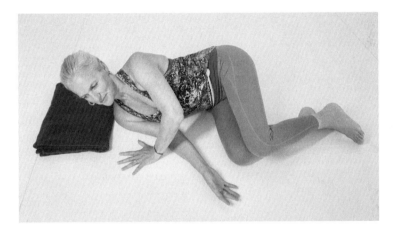

Figure 16: Coming out of the daily sequence

Cautionary notes

Stop exercising and talk to your doctor right away if you:
- get weaker, start losing your balance, or start falling
- have pain that gets worse
- have new heaviness, aching, tightness or other strange sensations in your arms or elsewhere
- have unusual swelling or any swelling gets worse

- have headaches, dizziness, blurred vision, new numbness or tingling in your arms or chest.

Avoid exercising if you:
- have a very low blood count
- have a fever of 38°C or above
- have an acute infection
- had surgery less than six weeks ago.

The A to Z of symptoms

Anxiety and 'scanxiety'

Being diagnosed with cancer challenges the assumption that we have control over our lives. Anxiety is a significant side effect and can be one of the most challenging of all. The human mind has the ability to imagine. When we worry our mind wanders or jumps forward into an imaginary future, and our thoughts are these little voices inside our head that just don't stop talking; they can talk non-stop. Thoughts are always busy, and our thoughts can create anxiety which you then might feel in your body as a sense of panic or a suffocating or scary feeling, because feelings are a response to something you are thinking or going through. **'Scanxiety'** is used to describe the anxiety induced by waiting for and having scans, an experience that is incredibly stressful, as is waiting for the results which might tell you that your cancer has shrunk, gone away or grown.

Your mind runs at a fast pace when you are anxious, and yoga can help you to get 'out of your head', give you a break from your thoughts and help you find some spaces between the sometimes-scary thoughts.

When you read this book, sit down and start to breathe: you are taking time out for *you*. This is precious time for you and your wellbeing. Putting yourself first isn't always easy but when you do take time for yourself, you are prioritising yourself and your wellbeing and starting to have a sense of taking back some control. You will be able to explore how different practices affect the way you feel. There isn't a one-size-fits-all in yoga so you can try different tools and see which ones work better for you. Which practice does actually give you some space between your thoughts? Which practice releases your physical body? Which one makes you feel calm and centred? How do you feel at the start of your practice? How do you feel at the end of your practice and what has changed or shifted? This is empowering.

If you can find something that makes you feel calmer and less anxious in a yoga practice, then you can use this in real life – when you are waiting for appointments, scan results or having treatment. Anytime you are aware of feeling anxious you can use the tools you learnt in this book to help you feel calmer or to observe your thoughts but not get hooked by them and bring yourself back to breathing or moving.

Understanding the nervous system

Our nervous system (NS) encompasses the central nervous system (CNS), the peripheral nervous system (PNS) and the autonomic nervous system (ANS). The **CNS** consists of the brain, 12 cranial nerves, the spinal cord and 31 pairs of spinal nerves. The nerves of the **PNS** connect the CNS to the organs, limbs and skin. If the peripheral nerves get damaged this can cause numbing or tingling or pain in the affected area (often the hands and feet) and is known as 'peripheral neuropathy'. We will explore how yoga can help improve balance and the small movements in the hands and feet in the chapter on Peripheral neuropathy (page 193).

In this chapter we will look more at the **ANS**, which is responsible for regulating involuntary body functions like digestion, heartbeat, blood flow and breathing. Anatomically and physiologically, we have two sides to our autonomic nervous system: the parasympathetic nervous system (PSNS) and the sympathetic nervous system (SNS). The side of the nervous system that is active and energy burning is the sympathetic side; it gets us up and ready to go. It also prepares us to fight, flee or freeze in threatening situations. It increases our heart and respiratory rate. Our blood pressure increases to get blood to vital organs and the muscles of our arms and legs so we can run from a situation or stay and fight. When we dial more into this part of the nervous system, inflammation is increased and the body burns more energy and releases free radicals (small particles that damage cells).

The soothing, relaxing and recharging side of the nervous system is the parasympathetic nervous system. Think of it as being like a parachute, slowing and calming us down. The heart rate and respiratory rate slow, blood pressure lowers, inflammation is reduced, and cells can be repaired. As the body rests and starts to digest fully, it is sometimes referred to as 'rest and digest mode'. This is the healing, nurturing and cleansing side of our nervous system. To have a healthy mind and body we need to balance the two sides of our autonomic nervous system.

When we change how we breathe we change the messages sent from the body's respiratory system to the brain. Powerful emotions can disrupt our breathing patterns. We gasp when we are in shock, breathe deeply in passionate moments and sob with grief. When you first heard the words 'you have cancer' your body and mind would have had an immediate response. You may have even held your breath or started to breathe erratically, and you would have gone into survival mode. Changes would have quickly happened to help you survive this attack. Perceived stress is the same as actual stress and stress changes the type of chemicals released by the body. The mind and the body are not separate. When we have feelings, emotions and thoughts we release neuropeptides. Positive neuropeptides such as serotonin and dopamine have a relaxing, positive and healthy effect on the body. We all know how great it feels when we wake up in the morning and the sky is blue and the sun is shining; we have positive thoughts about the day and this in return makes us feel good.

When we are stressed, we release the hormones cortisol and epinephrine (also called adrenaline). We need a certain amount of stress in our lives to get us up and out in our day. When we have to make a public speech or do something that puts us out of our comfort zone, then we will experience a feeling of stress. This kind of stress makes us feel awake, alive and excited. Sometimes our stress is triggered by an event, but if we allow our body to find a way to relax then it can return to homeostasis – or back to a sense of balance – and we are able to get back on with our day.

Using breathing to reduce stress

We now know that when we are repeatedly faced with stressful events, and we experience long-term or chronic stress, this weakens our immune system. We know that releasing stress helps strengthen it. Breathing is key to helping to release anxiety by bringing us into the present moment. When we are conscious of our breathing we are fully in the moment because we can't breathe in the past and we can't take a breath in the future. This means we are in this moment with whatever this moment brings.

Our overactive mind can be a wonderful thing, but it also can be limiting and scary. So, we need to take a break from thinking and bring ourselves into the present moment. If you feel anxious, just a few minutes of breathing can calm our mind. This allows us to be responsive and less reactive to the challenges around us.

There are many tools we can use to help bring us into the moment and it is about finding what works for you.

A simple wave breathing exercise

The next chapter will focus more on breathing but, to start taking back some control, find a comfortable sitting position where your spine feels long. This maybe in a chair or seated on some cushions on the floor. You could also do this lying down, but you might fall asleep – which might be just what you need!

If you are sitting, shift from side to side until you feel there is equal weight on both sitting bones. Your spine should feel long, and you should not be shifting forwards or backwards. As you breathe in, sense the wave-like motion of your breathing. Feel as you breathe in a wave rising and as you breathe out a wave falling. Some of us are more kinaesthetic, so you might physically sense the breath undulating through your body when you breathe in and out. A rising sensation as you breathe in, and a letting go or releasing sensation as you breathe out. You might be more visual and see or sense a wave on a lake as you breathe in and out. Or you might visualise your breathing as the waving of a flag or the undulation of sheets rippling on a washing line as they get blown with the wind. It doesn't matter how you sense, see or feel; just find your own way to experience this movement of breath in your own body.

Follow these steps:

- **Inhale** and sense or feel the wave rising.
- As you **exhale**, silently say to yourself '1'.
- **Inhale** and sense or feel the wave of breath rising.
- As you **exhale**, silently say to yourself '2'.
- **Inhale** and sense or feel the wave rising.
- As you **exhale** silently say '3'.
- **Inhale** and sense or feel the wave rising.
- As you **exhale** silently say '4'.
- … and continue in the same way, Incrementally counting upwards to '10' with each exhale and back down again to '1' (this takes about 2 minutes).

Then observe how you feel right now. What are the effects of the wave breath and counting? Did you lose count? Did your mind wander? It is totally normal for the mind to wander. The mind is just doing what the mind does. If you lose count because your mind got distracted, start back at the number '1' and begin again. Don't feel frustrated or annoyed. Turn up the corners of your mouth and smile. Let that smile radiate down through your body so you start the yoga practice of kindness and let go of any habitual patterns you have of judgement and labelling.

What are the effects of 2 minutes of conscious breathing? If you feel that this practice is beneficial then you can try this again. (Noting that if you count up to 10 and back down again 5 times this takes about 10 minutes.) If not, you can try one of the other meditation practices in this book to find one that resonates with you.

This wave breathing is a form of meditation because meditation is giving your mind something to focus on; here the focus is movement of breath and counting.

Point-to-point breathing in savasana pose

This is another breathing exercise to try in order to reduce stress and anxiety. First, get yourself into the savasana pose (see Figure 15, page 28).

- Establish relaxed, diaphragmatic breathing. Observe your breath.
- **Exhale** as if your breath is flowing from the crown of your head down to your toes. **Inhale** from your toes back to the crown of your head. Repeat 2–5 times.
- **Exhale** from your crown to your ankles; **inhale** from your ankles back to your crown and repeat 2–5 times.
- **Exhale** from your crown to your knees; **inhale** from your knees back to your crown. Repeat 2–5 times.
- **Exhale** down to the base of your spine; **inhale** from the base of your spine back to your crown. Repeat 2–5 times.
- **Exhale** down to your navel centre; **inhale** from your navel centre back to your crown. Repeat 2–5 times.
- **Exhale** down to your heart centre; **inhale** from your heart centre back to your crown. Repeat 2–5 times.
- **Exhale** down to your throat; **inhale** from your throat back to your crown. Repeat 2–5 times.
- **Exhale** to the centre between your eyebrows; **inhale** from the eyebrow centre back to your crown.
- Breathe back and forth between your crown and eyebrow centre, refining your breath and resting, repeating 5–10 times.
- Now reverse the order and descend, first to your throat centre, then to your heart centre, your navel centre… until you return to your toes.
- Finish by breathing out as if your whole body breathes. Let this **exhalation** flow downwards as if your breath is a wave flowing through the soles of your feet and on to infinity.

- Then, when **inhaling**, breathe as if your breath flows upwards through the crown of your head and on into infinity.
- You are lying in the centre of this infinite wave. Let your breathing remain deep and feel your breath as you relax your body and mind.

(Source: Sovik, 2006[1])

Each breath we take reminds us to be right here now. You might even contemplate how much more energy will be at your disposal when you are no longer wishing you were somewhere else doing something different.

Managing your thoughts

So, being diagnosed with cancer has highlighted that we are not in control of what life throws at us, but we can alter the way we interpret and respond to our stressful situations. This is not easy. Our thoughts can be like spam. The spam on our computer appeals to our fears and our greed. It highlights what we are missing and how, if only we were able to obtain something, then our lives would be better. Adverts remind us that we would be happier if we had a bigger house, a faster car or the right shampoo. When we worry we increase that spam in our brain.

What are you thinking about right now as you read this? The current thought that you are thinking now is totally under your control. The only thing any of us has under our control *is* our current thinking. If you follow that thought you are having, you will notice that it links to another thought and then another until you are miles away from your initial thought. Yoga can give us the opportunity to shave off the hooks from our thoughts. So, we can observe the thoughts that are bubbling to the surface, but we aren't getting hooked by them.

We all like to be heard and validated. When we are seen and heard we generally feel better about things, and so it is with our thoughts; we aren't pushing them away but learning to avoid intensifying them. Our mind seeks stimulation so notice your thoughts and, without pushing them away or trying to replace them with something else, can you just let them go with your exhale (outward breath). Not looking or hoping for something else. Allow each breath to come in and each exhale to let go.

Some moments in life *are* painful, sad and challenging and this is what might show up when you stop, start to consciously breathe and notice how busy your mind suddenly feels. These thoughts and feelings are not good or bad. They are not right or wrong. They just are as they are. So, notice if you tell yourself 'I shouldn't be thinking this' or if you judge your thoughts and give them the labels of 'right' and 'wrong'.

Paul Gilbert describes emotions as being 'sticky, as far as our thoughts are concerned.[2] Like magnets, they seem to pull our minds to them, and we find ourselves dwelling and ruminating on things that we are anxious, angry or depressed about. There's now a lot of evidence that ruminating on negative and unhappy subjects does us very little good... our thoughts and images can powerfully stimulate our bodies and the way they work.'

He reminds us that we only have to think about sexual imagery to see how thoughts can affect how we feel: 'So, think what we're doing to our brains when our minds go over and over things that we're angry, frightened or sad about. We're repeatedly stimulating the brain systems responsible for these negative thoughts and feelings, which isn't conducive to our wellbeing or our happiness.'

I often hear that there is a pressure to try to be positive. Sometimes this is because you are caretaking others and need to keep on a brave face to look after others and how they are responding to your diagnosis. It is normal to experience negativity, and we can't be happy all the time. The yoga sutras, the ancient texts on yoga, speak of **'santosha'** meaning contentment – being content with what is and not needing to fix our change, as much as we might desperately want to change and fix. This might be by taking baby steps and not looking too far forward into the future but instead just taking each moment as it is.

We can observe our feelings of anger, loss or disappointment but we want to move beyond those feelings so that they can't influence us and our daily lives. When we do try to get rid of, or judge, those thoughts and say, 'I shouldn't feel or think that,' then they just will come back and seem magnified.

Have you ever woken up first thing and not been sure where you were or what day of the week it was? For a moment you have a sense of 'no thought' and then your mind starts to awaken, and you remember what day it is, where you are and what you have to do today. Our mind swings like a pendulum from the moment we awake. It swings into the past, looking back or rehashing things we have already done, and then it swings forward to the future to things that haven't yet happened and may never happen. It's a safety thing. Our mind is looking forward to events, then looking back to see if we have had any experience previously. Is there something we did or didn't do before? If it was positive, we might try to repeat something we did in the past or try to learn from it if it was a mistake.

Our mind has evolved for scarcity, not abundance, so it has a natural negativity bias. In prehistoric times we needed to look out for dangers as we searched for food and shelter, focusing on negative things that might affect our survival. So, anxiety, scanxiety (see page 33), anger and other similar emotions are normal responses to life and essential to our survival. Fear is a survival response so we can accept it as one of our experiences, be aware of how we are feeling and say hello to our fear. We can acknowledge that our fear helps us to survive and that it is part of our life experience. It can feel easier to cope with fear if we can befriend it as a necessary part of what you are going through. Unpleasant experiences *are* part of life, and this is part of being human. If we go round and round and round with our thoughts, we end up revolving and not evolving, so how can we observe what is going on, acknowledge and befriend the thoughts as just our thoughts, and not let them intensify and give our mind something else to focus on?

The negativity bias explains why we are Teflon to compliments (they don't stick) and Velcro to insults (they adhere to us and stay with us). The neuropsychologist Dr Rick Hanson has looked at brain activity and points out that the amygdala, the brain's alarm system, dedicates two-thirds of its neutrons to processing negative experiences.[3] You can receive lots of compliments and one negative comment and that negative comment is the one that sticks with you and goes around and around in your head. That pendulum of our mind swings forwards into the future and back into the past, trying to make sense of it – swinging into the past to search for similar experiences so we can see how we dealt with them before. What did we do that we can use in the future to protect ourselves? Or what mistakes did we make in the past that we don't want to repeat in the future?

Furthermore, our brain doesn't know the difference between a perceived threat and a real threat; so, with a cancer diagnosis, we live in a state of arousal with many perceived threats. Fear can make us feel smaller, protecting our vulnerable areas as we drop our head, lift our shoulders, round our backs and close off our hearts. When we are fearful and not breathing fully, we can get cut off from receiving essential energy, but when we are excited about living, we invite energy into our body. You might have felt this when you have experienced something amazing like an incredible view in nature or the excitement of your football team scoring a goal.

Meditation

There is no one-size-fits-all and there are many ways to quieten the mind, but the first thing you might notice when you start to practise yoga is how loud your mind is. Indeed, it may appear as though you have even more thoughts and this might make you want to stop the practice, especially if the thoughts you observe are challenging, upsetting or distressing.

Our thoughts can be like a fast-moving river. This river may have rapids and rocks and it can pull us under the water with its currents and we may feel sometimes as though we can't get our heads above the water. The stream of thoughts can also pull us into directions that we don't want to go or even in directions we had no idea we were going in. When we find some tools to help us calm our mind and become present, we can find ourselves on the banks of the river. We can see the fast-moving water of thoughts and see how they swirl around, but we aren't getting pulled along by them or pulled under. We can become an observer but not a participant. Easier said than done and I think the key word here would be 'practise' because the more we practise, like any new skill we try to learn, the more skilled we will become and the easier it will be. Meditation is a practice, something that we can keep coming back to – a practice to be present with this moment, to feel it, to know it and to fully experience it. To meditate is to listen with a receptive and non-judgemental heart.

Meditating on anything one chooses that is elevating is the pathway to removing the obstacles to self-realisation.[4]

All you need for meditation is a focus for your mind. This might be your breath, a word, a mantra or a phrase. You might have an affirmation that you feel would be helpful and supportive, like 'calm and centred' or 'healthy and strong'. It could also be a physical sensation, a flower, a candle or a fixed gaze. You also need a non-judgemental attitude about your 'performance'. As you sit you start to be aware or notice thoughts bubbling up. You can observe your thoughts as they arise, noticing what is coming up during your practice, accepting what is arising and not trying to suppress it or push it away. Instead of following your thoughts, come back to following your breath or a mantra.

When we meditate, we notice that our minds are constantly distracted. Notice the wandering of thoughts and gently and kindly bring your mind back to the task of breathing, or whatever your focus might be. It is natural to wonder if you are doing it 'right' and this is understandable, but it is a distraction. Observe the distraction with a hint of a smile and compassionately and kindly bring your attention back to the task of breathing or following a focus.

Body scans

A body scan is one of the most accessible meditative practices and involves bringing your attention to your body, noticing sensations as you mentally scan your body from your head to your toes or from toes to head.

When you become still, your body temperature can drop so it might be good to have a blanket to cover you. You might need to raise your knees to release tension in your lower back or find a position that you are comfortable in. As you begin to shift your awareness through areas of your body there is no need to move anything. You might mentally repeat the name of the part of the body or just let your awareness rest there. You might start with your feet, then ankles, calves, shins, backs of knees, thighs, pelvis, lower back, middle back, upper back, chest, shoulders, arms, hands, neck, jaw, mouth, cheeks, nose, eyes and forehead.

As you breathe in, you can start to imagine your breath starting at your toes like a wave and travelling up your body and out of the crown of your head; then, as you breathe out, your breath sweeps back down your body from the top of your head down to your toes.

For a more detailed body scan see the chapter on 'Referred pain' – page 201.

Breathing

As outlined in the last chapter, 'Anxiety and scanxiety', the quickest way we can change how we feel is by changing the way we breathe. Just by bringing mindful attention to your breathing you become present in this moment right now. We can't breathe in the future or breathe in the past, so by observing your breath right now you are brought into the present moment.

When we are anxious, our sympathetic nervous system is dominant, and our breathing is typically shorter and shallower. Our shoulders may rise up and down as we inhale and exhale. Through some simple breathing techniques, we can use our breath to soothe the nervous system, stimulate the parasympathetic nervous system and induce the relaxation response.

Three-part breathing

To start consciously being aware of your breath you might want to find a comfortable position lying down. This might make it easier to feel your breath moving into your body as gravity will help you to feel what is being explored in this exercise. You might need some support, a rolled-up blanket under your knees or a blanket under your head so your neck feels long (see Figure 17).

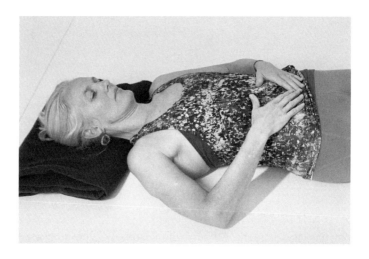

Figure 17 Supporting your head with a blanket; observing the
movement of breath in your belly

Take a moment to scan your body. You might start at your toes and slowly work your way up to your ankles, calves, shins, knees, thighs, pelvis, belly, lower back, middle back, upper back. Then, letting your chest soften, arms, hands and throat. Soften your lower jaw, gums and teeth, allow your tongue to broaden and soften and release your upper jaw, gums and teeth. Feel the breath in your nostrils. Maybe you can sense that the breath feels warmer when you breathe out and cooler when you breathe in? Soften your eyes and the skin across your forehead.

Notice what it feels like to be in your body at this moment. It may be different to how you felt yesterday or the last time you had time to stop and observe yourself.

Observing breathing into the physical body

As you start to breathe into your body, you may notice areas of tension – maybe areas you are guarding, areas where you have had surgery or where your body has compensated to protect vulnerable areas. You may notice imbalances in your body. See if you can notice, without judgement, the tighter areas, or parts of your body that are tense. Without labelling anything as good or bad, just start following the air as it travels in and out through your nostrils. (If you are congested, part your lips and breathe in through your mouth.)

Breath ratios

Notice the ratio of your breathing. Count your breath in and your breath out. Just notice what your natural ratio is, not judging it but just noticing.

Start to work towards an even inhale and exhale. Try not to force your breath ratios or to have ratios that are too challenging as this might start to create a feeling of stress.

As the breath affects the nervous system, so your breath can start to have an effect on your body. The quickest way to balance the nervous system is to breathe in and out to the same count. So, if you breathe in for 2 you breathe out for 2; if you breathe in for 3, breathe out for 3; in for 4, out for 4. It doesn't matter what your count is, only that your breathing in and out is even.

Concentrate on exhaling completely to get rid of stale air. Carbon dioxide (CO_2) is heavier than air and hangs out in the bottom of your lungs. Focus on exhaling from the bottom up. At the end of your exhale, you could squeeze the stale air out like toothpaste. We can only breathe in fully if we can breathe out fully. Alan Hymes, in *The Science of Breath*, says that the best breathing practice for everyday relaxed functioning is diaphragmatic breathing: 'Here lung expansion is focused on the lower, gravity dependent areas of the lungs where oxygen exchange can proceed more efficiently,' by which he means that more oxygen moves from the lungs into the bloodstream.[1]

Put your hands onto your belly and feel it rise on the inhale and fall on the exhale (see Figure 17 – page 44). Have you been scared to move this area of your body? Is this an area of surgery or treatment? You might be breathing into areas that you have been avoiding moving into? Can you feel your breath starting to soothe and massage your body from the inside out?

The diaphragm, which is our main breathing muscle, should move when we breathe in and out. The central tendon of the diaphragm contracts when we breathe in and draws down; this pushes down onto the abdominal cavity and the abdominal organs get pressed and the belly moves. So, when we are breathing fully, we are using our diaphragm and we will feel some movement in the belly. This helps to improve circulation by compressing and gently massaging our internal organs.

Let each breath flow naturally into the next. Can you breathe evenly into both sides of your belly? Observe if your breath gets stuck anywhere and direct your breath into areas that feel they aren't receiving breath. Just observe the breath in your belly. Don't judge how you breathe; just observe.

Breathe in, belly rises. Breathe out, belly falls.

Is this what is happening to you? Sometimes when we are stressed, we reverse-breathe, which means our belly draws in and up on inhale and presses out on exhale. If you notice that your breathing pattern is different, then just being aware of this is the first stage of change. See if you can soften your belly so that it receives breath as you breathe in; this way you start to break the reverse-breathing pattern and start to focus on 'full-body', or 'three-part', breathing.

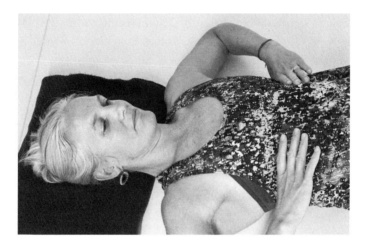

Figure 18: Observing the movement of breath in your ribs

Then take your hands to your ribs (see Figure 18). Feel your ribs expand as you inhale, and your fingers move apart. As you exhale feel your ribs soften and your fingers move closer together. A little bit like the opening of an umbrella, the ribs move outwards as you inhale and then close inwards as you exhale. Breathe wide into your ribs and feel the expansive quality of the breath and then, as you breathe out, feel a sensation of letting go.

Then take your hands to the top of your chest and breathe fully into your collar bones (see Figure 19). Feel the breath in the top part of the chest expanding as you inhale and releasing and softening as you exhale. Again, sense the massaging quality of the breath from the inside of the body out. Breathing into areas of the chest that feel tight, restricted or where you might have felt scared to move.

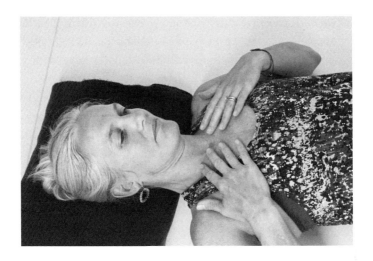

Figure 19: Feeling your breath in the top part of your chest

Then keep one hand on your heart and one hand on your belly. Breathe into your heart and radiate love from it to other areas of your body that you feel need some TLC (tender loving care) (see Figure 20).

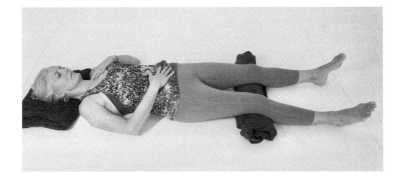

Figure 20: Breathing into the heart and radiating love to other areas of the body

This breathing exercise is what is called three-part breathing – beginning with the belly moving, the ribs expanding and the chest lifting on inhale and the reverse on exhale. However, there is also a version taught by T K V Desikachar (and a style of yoga called Viniyoga) where this order is reversed (see his book, *The Heart of Yoga*:

developing a personal practice[2]): first the upper chest is lifted, then the lower ribs are elevated to the side, and finally the belly rises. There is no right or wrong way to breathe and you might just find that one version resonates more with you or works better for you.

I have some students who say that they breathe better when they imagine breathing into the back of their body. They can feel their breath move into their upper back, middle back and lower back as they draw the breath down into the lower lobes of their lungs. In fact, in Desikachar's book he says that breathing into the belly first can 'inhibit the expansion of the chest and consequently the spine is not extended enough' and that the rising action of the chest gives room for the diaphragm to move freely. So, it is worth trying the breathing technique of breathing chest, ribs then abdomen if you find that breathing into abdomen, ribs and then chest more challenging. When lying down you might also feel your breath actually breathing out into your yoga mat, floor or bed.

Supine twist

It is common under stress that our shoulders move as we use secondary breathing muscles to get more breath into our lungs. If you find that your shoulders are moving up and down as you breathe in and out, you could try the breathing practice in a supine twist (see Figure 21).

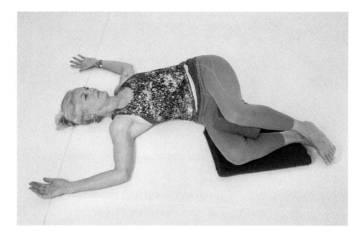

Figure 21: The supine twist

Support your legs with a blanket or cushion and maybe place a cushion or yoga block in between your shins or thighs so that you keep your knees hip distance apart and your lower back feels happy. Stretch your arms out in line with your shoulders and, with your knees bent, take your knees over to one side. If this is too much of a stretch on your chest or shoulders, then change the angle of your arms or try bending your elbows. You want to feel that your chest is open but not in any pain. Keep your arms symmetrical so your stronger arm might lower to be at the same angle as your arm with limited range of motion if this is the case for you.

Then follow the three-part breathing exercise outlined previously. The twist should help to keep your shoulders fixed and relaxed so you can feel the breath first in your belly, then in your ribs and then in your chest.

Lengthening the exhale to calm

When we breathe in, we energise our body, stimulating the sympathetic nervous system (SNS) (fight or flight): if you feel your pulse, it will quicken when you breathe in. When we breathe out, we stimulate the parasympathetic nervous system (PSN) (rest and digest): if you feel your pulse, it will slow when you breathe out. Therefore, it makes sense to start to lengthen your exhale as a way of calming down your body and mind.

If you find counting your breaths a useful tool, you might continue with counting and see if you can make your exhale a count longer than your inhale. It may not even be a full count but just a nano second longer than the inhale. Remember, it is a practice and so the more we practise consciously breathing the better we will become at breathing.

Sound

We can also use sound to help to lengthen the breath out and to focus our mind. When we hum, the sound and its vibrations fill our body and help to quieten our constantly busy and chattering mind. Take a deep breath in and, as you exhale, hum. Repeat this a few more times. Then stop and observe. Notice if the humming made the exhale longer. Did it make you focus more on the breath and draw your awareness inwards? Did it bring you more into the present moment?

Breathing with a hum or a sound stimulates the vagus nerve, which is the main pathway of the parasympathetic nervous system. The vocal cords contract to make this humming sound and this resistance creates a vibrations that soothe the nervous system. Cats do this naturally when they purr.

The vibrations stimulate the vagus nerve and the PSN as well as the organs and tissues. Sound waves travel through water and, as our organs are made up of water, then we can sense the vibrations massaging through and around them.

Nose breathing

Why is breathing through the nose so beneficial? When we breathe in through our nose, the breath is stirred up by turbinates in our nostrils. Swami Rama, Ballentine and Hymes describe these turbinates as 'seashell-like bulges' that create turbulence and, as the air circulates over these bulges, it becomes warm and moist.[1] The hairs in the nostrils also filter and clean our breath. Breathing through the nose releases nitric oxide, which is necessary to increase carbon dioxide in the blood which in turn releases oxygen. James Nestor's awesome book *Breath* explains how the 'sinuses release a huge boost of nitric oxide, a molecule that plays an essential role in increasing circulation and delivering oxygen into cells…nasal breathing alone can boost nitric oxide six-fold which is one of the reasons we can absorb about 18% more oxygen by just breathing through the nose'.[3]

The nose also slows and deepens the breath and as a result it fills the lungs more effectively from top to bottom.

Congested nose

However, if you are at all congested, then it is better to breathe through the mouth than not breathe at all! Try breathing through partly closed lips as you inhale and exhale, as breathing through an open mouth can be dehydrating.

If you are congested, you can also try this technique to unblock your nasal passages:
- Take your right hand into your left armpit and your left hand into your right armpit.
- Breathe into your hands as they sit in your armpits and feel the gentle pressure of breath into your ribs, armpits and hands. The pressure of the right hand should help clear the left nostril and the pressure of the left hand can help clear the right nostril.

- Breathe smoothly and evenly into your hands for 2–3 minutes and see if this has helped to release any congestion.

If breathing is challenging due to tumours pressing on airwaves, then you might have to adapt some of the poses so that you are able to breathe. With lung cancer you could try focusing on breathing into your belly avoiding focusing on your lungs. It might be more comfortable lying over a bolster and being slightly propped up. Try focusing more on your **exhale** than your inhale if you find it hard to get breath into your body. Think of your breath as starting with your exhale and, if you can breathe out fully and let go, you create a vacuum for breath to just naturally get drawn into your body. We can only fully breathe in when we learn to fully breathe out.

Lying down can make it harder to breathe so if this is something you experience then maybe prop yourself up on blankets or bolsters for breath work done lying on your back.

Avoid any breath counts that are straining. Find breath counts that work for you. Especially when you are adding on movement to your practice.

- For energising alternate nostril breathing techniques see the chapter on 'Fatigue' (page 83).
- For balanced breathing techniques see the chapter on 'Nausea' (see page 165).
- For calming alternate nostril breathing see the chapter 'ZZZZZ – sleep and insomnia' (page 267).
- For cooling breathing techniques see the chapter 'Hot flushes' (page 97).

Chemo brain

According to Macmillan Cancer Support, 'Changes in memory or concentration and the ability to think clearly during cancer treatment are often called cancer-related cognitive changes (CRCC) or chemo brain'.[1] Chemo brain can make it difficult to efficiently process information and is a diagnosable condition that may be caused by the cancer, by chemotherapy treatment or by secondary conditions like anaemia. You might be finding it hard to remember things or feel foggy, distracted and/or disorganised, and this can be incredibly frustrating.

Fatigue and sleep problems can worsen chemo brain symptoms so following the sequences in the chapter 'Zzzzz – sleep and insomnia' (page 267) can help you relax and calm before bed which can in turn help with sleep. This will also help ease stress. Yoga can help to elevate our mood and give us a better feeling of wellbeing, which can also help with symptoms.

In 2014 there was more positive research on yoga and 'cognitive problems' for breast cancer survivors. In a randomised controlled trial, it was found that participants in a 12-week Hatha yoga program vs. a control group witnessed a 3% improvement in their cognitive ability. Furthermore, those that practised most frequently (vs. less frequently) reported better improvement.[2] Another study has shown that breast cancer patients who exercised had reduced inflammation and 'chemo brain'.[3]

Yoga techniques to help improve concentration

Hakini mudra

A useful mudra you could try is the **hakini mudra** where you bring the fingertips of each hand together like a tee pee or tent (see Figure 22). Gertrud Hirschi in *Mudras – yoga in your hands*, states that this finger position has been well-researched and promotes the cooperation between the right- and left-brain hemispheres.[4] It is said, according to Gertrud, to 'open access to the right hemisphere, which is where the memory is stored'. She advises taking the tip of the tongue to the roof of the mouth behind the front teeth whilst inhaling and letting the tongue fall on exhaling when your hands are in this mudra position.

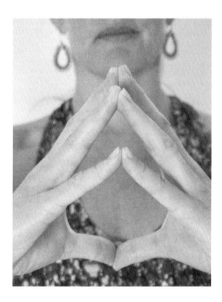

Figure 22 The hakini mudra

Sat nam meditation

The Kundalini yoga tradition has a meditation that is said to help to stimulate brain activity and relax the nerves. The US-based Alzheimer's Research and Prevention Foundation recommends this to improve cognition and activate parts of the brain that are central to memory.[5] I find that, by focusing on the chant, the movement of my fingers and the repetition, that I am so distracted I can get a break from thinking. This quietens my mind from my thoughts and gives me a sense of calm.

The sounds in this meditation come from the mantra **sat nam** which means 'my true essence'.

- Take your thumb to your index fingertip and mentally say 'saa'
- Then move your thumb to your middle fingertip and mentally say 'taa'
- Then move your thumb to your ring fingertip and mentally say 'naa'
- Then move your thumb to your little fingertip and mentally say 'maa'.

Repeat in this sequence and, if you feel comfortable, you may want to sing the chant 'saa taa naa maa' out loud for a few rounds.

Next, whisper the chant for a few rounds and then come back to mentally chanting as you move your fingers.

You can practise this mudra and mantra for as long as you feel comfortable. You might want to end with a few minutes just seated and breathing before you start to slowly move back into your day.

Varying your yoga poses

To keep our brain stimulated it is good to vary our practices, to try things that challenge us, maybe that challenge our sense of balance or make us look at things in a different way. If you normally do poses that are static, try doing them dynamically, moving in and out with your breath. Here are a few other suggestions of ways you can change your practice to keep stimulating the brain.

Diagonal steps

- From the front of your mat, inhale and step your right foot back to the right side of the mat. Then exhale and step your right foot back to the front of the mat.
- Then inhale and step your right foot to the left side of the mat (so you are stepping diagonally) and then exhale and step your right foot back to the front of the mat.
- Repeat this a few times with your right foot, varying the side of the mat you are stepping back to.

- Then repeat the moves, this time stepping with your left foot to the left side of the mat.

Walking your mat

Starting at one end of your mat, place your feet onto one of its long edges and walk forward along that edge to the other end of the mat. Then walk backwards along the long edge to the other end of your mat. When this starts to become easy, try this with your eyes closed.

Arm circles

Try circling your arms both going in the same direction.

Then try uncoupling your limbs and circle one arm one way and the other in the opposite direction. Then try reversing it.

Tree pose

Try a tree pose balancing on one leg with the other foot resting above or below the knee. Then try it with your arms behind your back, or with your eyes closed (stay close to a wall!) or try a **dynamic tree pose**.

- **Inhale** and raise your arms and your right knee, taking your foot to your shin (see Figure 23).
- **Exhale** and lower your arms and your foot (see Figure 24).
- **Inhale** and raise your arms and your left knee, taking your foot to your shin (see Figure 25).
- **Exhale** and lower your arms and your foot as before (see Figure 24).

Additional warm-up moves

When practising the warm-up series described in the 'Introduction' (Figures 1 to 16) you could also try reaching opposite arm to opposite leg as you draw your knee in. Just changing our habits and usual patterns keeps us more alert and stops us moving on autopilot. If you make mistakes and it is challenging, try to smile and let the essence of the smile radiate down through your body. Balance is a skill we can learn and relearn.

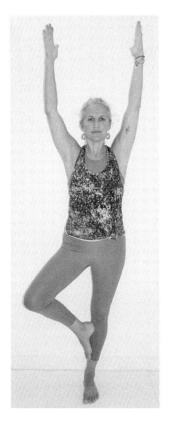

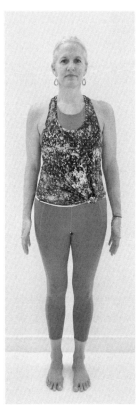

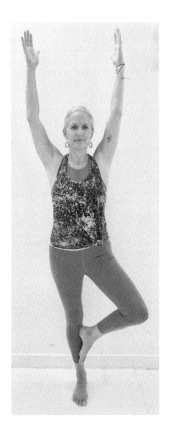

Figure 23: Dynamic tree pose (a) raising your arms and right knee

Figure 24: Dynamic tree pose (b) lowering arms and foot

Figure 25: Dynamic tree pose (c) raising your arms and left knee

Colostomy, ostomy, ileostomy and yoga with a stoma

Everything in this book is suitable for someone living with a stoma, whether semi-permanent or permanent. As with any surgery, you would want to be about six weeks post-surgery with all surgical incisions healed before trying any of the exercises. I have worked with many students with stomas, and they are able to practise yoga and have found benefits from bringing breath and movement into the areas of the body they have guarded or protected.

If you have a stoma, then I would highly recommend reading Sarah Russell's *The Bowel Cancer Recovery Toolkit*,[1] which looks at exercising and living with a stoma. Sarah's book explores extensively what can be done even a few days after surgery and also what exercises should be avoided or included only when strength is built back. Leslie Howard's book *Pelvic Liberation* is another must-read for expert guidance on releasing, stretching and strengthening your pelvic floor.[2] I share with you information that I have learnt from training with Leslie.

This chapter explores how we can release tension that may be being held in the pelvis from the trauma of surgery. Healthy muscles have a full range of motion. Muscles that are held tight are not necessarily strong muscles and, because they are tight, they are not moving through their full range of motion. So first we will look at releasing tight muscles, because surgery may have restricted flexibility in the abdominal area. Then we will look at how to find a neutral spine so that we can move safely through other sequences in this book and use our deep core muscles to support us and help us to build strength.

Releasing tight muscles

- Start by lying supine (on your back) on your mat.
- Place a bolster or 3–4 folded towels under your sacrum. Your sacrum is the flat part of your lower back where your pelvis is, so not your lumbar, which is the part of your lower back where you can feel your spine.
- You might lift your pelvis away from your support for a moment and then lengthen your tailbone away from your face to lengthen your spine (see Figure 26).

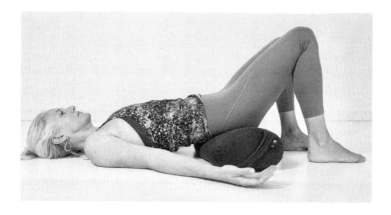

Figure 26: Lifting your pelvis and lengthening your tailbone

When we elevate the pelvis like this, we take the weight of the organs away from the pelvic floor and it makes it easier to sense or feel our pelvic floor. The pelvic floor moves with our breathing, and it mirrors the diaphragm (our main breathing muscle). When we breathe in, the pelvic floor broadens and when we breathe out, the pelvic floor domes upwards towards our heart.

As you breathe in and out in this position, notice the pressure changes in your body and where you might observe the breath moving into your body. Can you feel breath moving down your body or does it get stuck anywhere? If your body has experienced trauma, then it might be harder to breathe into these areas. There are areas we might be guarding or protecting. Also notice if you can breathe in evenly on both sides. If you sense that your breath is not moving into a particular area of your body, can you start to direct your breath into that area? When we breathe in, we draw energy into our body so can you start to direct that energy (or prana) into those areas that feel stuck or that you might have been nervous of moving or stretching?

Then try adding the **apana vayu mudra** to see if it helps to release tension held in your belly (see Figure 27). 'Vayu' refers to the winds or the five various movements of energy in the body. 'Prana' is a forward-moving energy and 'apana' is a downward-moving energy that we need for eliminating and detoxifying. Because of the focus on downward-moving energy, this mudra might help to release tightness in your pelvis and pelvic floor.

Bring your index fingers to the base of your thumb.

Then bring your ring and middle finger to the tip of your thumb.

(This mudra is not advisable if you have diarrhoea.)

As you bring your hands into this gesture, does it change anything about your breath moving into your body? Is it easier to breathe or are you aware of breath more in your upper body or lower body? If it is harder to breathe, then let go of the mudra.

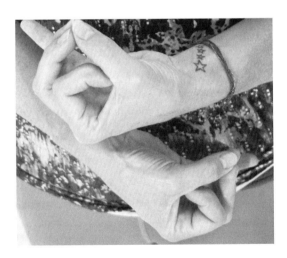

Figure 27: The apana vayu mudra

Bringing the spine into a neutral position

Our deep core muscles are the pelvic floor, diaphragm, transverse abdominis and multifidus muscles and they are more accessible when our spine is in neutral. When we start to round our spine to use our core, then we are making our superficial tummy muscles, like the rectus abdominus, work harder (our six-pack muscles).

- Keep your spine neutral so you feel your rib cage on the mat and your pelvis on the bolster.
- Bring your hands to your belly and as you **exhale** make a 'sssshhhhhhh' sound; exhale all the air out and you will feel your belly draw in and slightly up.
- Observe the natural movement of pelvic floor and diaphragm drawing in and up towards your heart on exhale.
- We want to use this movement to help us build strength in our deep core muscles, so next time you exhale and firm your belly, keep the shape of your spine (not rounding it or letting your belly pop up to the ceiling) and draw your right knee towards you (see Figure 28).
- **Inhale** and then **exhale**, firming your belly as you lower your right foot back down to the floor. The hardest part is to keep your belly firm and not arch your lower back just before your foot touches the floor. Try to keep a neutral spine so you aren't rounding or collapsing in the lower back.
- **Exhale**, firming your belly and lift your left knee towards you.
- **Inhale** and then **exhale**, lowering your left foot back down.

If this felt really challenging then you might continue moving just on your exhale. If you want more of a challenge:

- **Exhale** and lift your right foot and draw your knee in towards you without changing the shape of your spine.
- **Inhale** and lower your right foot back down.
- **Exhale** lifting your left foot away from the floor and left knee towards you.
- **Inhale** and lower your left foot back down.
- You might also try exploring what it feels like to lift both knees away from the floor as you **exhale** and then **inhale** as you lower them both back down.

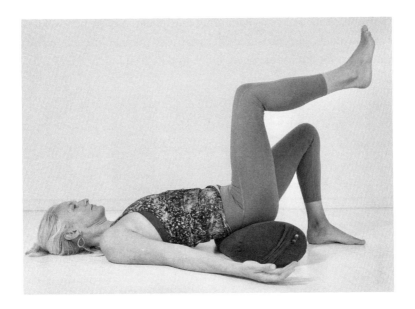

Figure 28: Keeping the spine neutral while engaging the core

You should feel your lower belly working and the strengthening of your deep core muscles. **However,** if you find that you feel it in your lower back, take the props out and move to the natural and neutral spine exercise described below and then maybe come back to the bolster or blankets.

Natural or neutral spine

Let's explore what a natural or neutral spine actually feels like.
- Press down into your feet to lift your bottom away from the bolster/blankets and move them out of the way. Rest your lower back on the mat and explore the natural curves of your spine.
- As you **inhale** let your pubic bone move away from your head and as you **exhale** draw your pubic bone towards your head. Feel how your lower back presses into the mat (flexion) – see Figure 29.
- **Inhale** and move your pubic bone away from you and feel how you get some space at your lower back (lumbar) – see Figure 30.
- **Exhale** and move your pubic bone towards you and feel how your lower back rounds towards the floor.

These pelvic rocking exercises help bring movement into the pelvis but also make us aware of how our spine can round (flex) towards the mat or curve away from the mat (extend). Can you find somewhere in the middle (see Figure 31)?

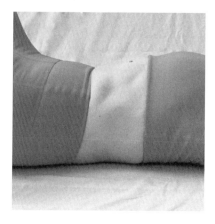

Figure 29: Lower back pressing into the mat

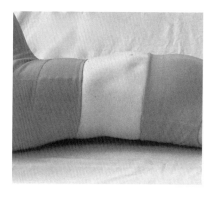

Figure 30: Arching of the lower back

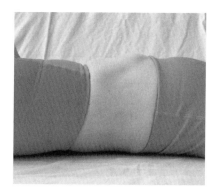

Figure 31: Keeping a natural curve in the lower back

The natural curves of the spine, or 'neutral' spine, is where the spine feels long and flat, but we know it isn't flat because it has its natural curves. **Neutral spine** is something we will come back to throughout this book as it is **a key component of practising yoga safely**. When we are working with the natural curves of our spine our spine is stronger and we are able to incorporate the deep core muscles and use them to help support us.

Leg muscles

Opening the inner thighs

When we stretch our inner thigh muscles, or adductors, this can help to lengthen the second layer of the pelvic floor.
- Find the natural curves of your spine.
- **Exhale**, firm your belly and lift your feet away from the floor.
- Hold onto your right knee/shin with your right hand and left knee/shin with your left hand.
- Keeping the natural curves of your spine, let your knees travel away from you and away from each other. Your legs will look like a short V shape (see Figure 32).
- Notice if you have become heavier on one side of your pelvis than on the other. Can you create a sense of balance in the pelvis?
- Then as you **exhale**, firm your belly and start to straighten your right leg without shifting to the right (see Figure 33).
- **Inhale** and re-bend your right knee.
- **Exhale** and straighten your left leg.
- **Inhale** re-bend your knee.

Continue 2–3 more times on each side. You might want to stay in the pose and hold for a few breaths or continue moving dynamically. Can you breathe all the way down to your pelvic floor?

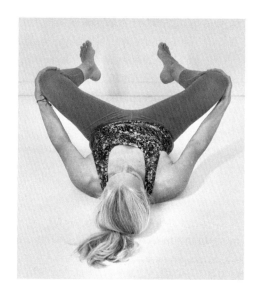

Figure 32: Opening the inner thighs to a V-shape

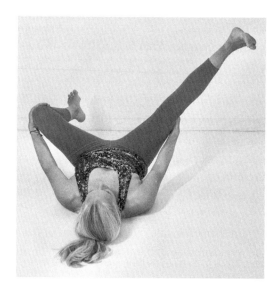

Figure 33: Straightening your leg

Hamstring stretch

Releasing the hamstring (the muscles that run down the back of the upper leg) can help lengthen the first and third layers of the pelvic floor:

- Find the natural curves of your spine.
- Draw your right knee in without changing the shape of your lower back. If you pull your knee in too close you will feel how your spine rounds to the floor, so then slightly press your thigh away from you to get the natural curve of your spine.
- Place a strap or scarf around the ball of your right foot, where it meets your arch.
- Extend the foot up into the strap towards the ceiling.
- Keeping the neutral spine, use the strap to draw your thighbone down into your pelvis. If this is challenging on your chest or armpits, you can try crossing the strap in front of your leg, as shown in Figure 34. Widen your arms and bend your elbows resting them on the mat so your chest feels open and spacious (see Figure 34).
- You can keep your left knee bent or, if it doesn't cause pain in your lower back, then you can straighten your left leg out along the mat.
- Press your left foot into an imaginary wall or you can even position yourself so that your foot can press into an actual wall. The wall will give you some feedback on what is happening in your left leg. It will help you discern

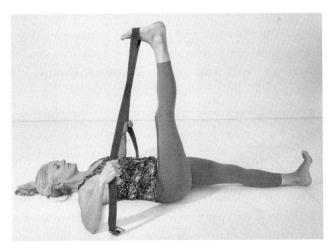

Figure 34: Using a strap to release the hamstring

whether your leg is actually straight, or if your toes turn out and your leg is externally rotating.

- Roll your inner thigh to the floor. Try to keep your toes pointing up to the ceiling and straighten your leg by pressing the top of your thigh to the floor and not your knee. If this causes any discomfort in your lower back, then re-bend your left knee and place the foot back onto the floor.
- Stay here for about 1-2 minutes, breathing and feeling breath move into your upper back, middle back and down into your lower back.
- Exhale out from the belly.
- To come out, bend both knees. Bring your feet back down to the mat.
- Pause to observe the differences in your right and left leg. I also find if I straighten out my legs, my right leg now feels much longer than the left leg. You can explore if this is something you feel?
- Repeat on the left side.

Figure-of-four

- Bend both knees and, keeping your neutral spine position, draw your right knee in and cross your right ankle over your left thigh.
- Flex your right foot.
- As you **exhale**, firm your belly and draw your left knee in towards you.
- Keeping the weight in your sacrum/pelvic area, take hold of the back of your left leg (see Figure 11 on page 25). I find if I interlace my fingers this allows my chest and shoulders to relax, but if this is a strain on your arms/chest area, then you can use the strap or a scarf to lengthen your arms. Another option is to elevate the floor by placing a block under your left foot.
- Stay for 1–2 minutes and then change sides.

Other poses to try

Two other poses in this book that can help to open up the pelvic floor and relax the abdomen are described in the chapter on 'Digestion': the restorative pose, **legs-over-a-chair** (page 155), to release the psoas, and the **supta baddha konasana** (page 163) to open up the belly and groin area. Also see the **circular lunges** in the chapter on 'Menopause' (page 157).

Cramps

Leg cramps are a painful tightening of the muscles in the leg, ankle or foot and can be caused by some hormone drugs, peripheral neuropathy, certain chemotherapy or immunotherapy treatments and radiation therapy to the hips and legs.

We look at wonderful ways to open up the feet in the 'Peripheral neuropathy' (page 193) and 'Joint pain' (page 109) chapters, but the following exercise to relieve cramp in your lower leg is a favourite one for my students and is often requested in classes, I am grateful to Leslie Howard for introducing me to this great release.[1] You don't need any props and you could even do this lying in your bed. It is a massage that helps to find any tight points and releases the connective tissue in the calves. Because you are doing it by yourself you can spend as long as you want on the massage.

- Bend both knees and then place the back of your right knee on top of your left knee so you feel the very top of your right calf pressing on top of your left knee (see Figure 35).
- Relax your right foot and then, staying in situ to begin with, start to move your right leg forward and back in place. You should feel a massaging-like pressure at the top of your right calf.
- Then, slowly moving at your own pace, start to move down the centre of your calf until you *slowly* get down towards your heel. When it starts to feel more fibrous and less like your fleshy calf muscle you will be feeling the beginning of the tendon that attaches the calf to the heel.
- Once you get to that point start to move back up your calf muscle, but this time moving up more to the outside of the calf. This can sometimes feel tighter, or you find some 'interesting' points of tension as you might start to feel the muscles besides the calf (gastrocnemius) called fibularis.

- Taking your time, slowly massage back up to the back of the knee. Once you have finished, uncross your legs and straighten them both out.
- Then pause. Notice your breath moving into your body. Is it easier to breathe into the side of the calf you have massaged? Do your legs feel different left to right? Does your right leg feel more awake or alive? Take a moment to observe the effects of releasing the connective tissue in your calf. The body is connected by this tissue so you may be aware of changes elsewhere in your body.
- It is good to massage both calves at the same time, so now repeat this exercise with the left leg.

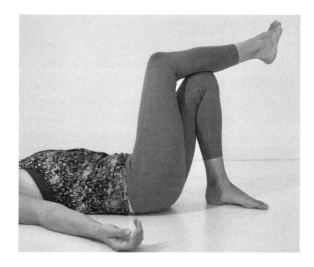

Figure 35: Right knee on top of left knee for cramp massage

Digestive problems and discomfort

Treatment for cancer targets fast-growing cells like cancer cells, but we also have fast-growing cells in our digestive system and so side effects may include feeling sick (nausea), diarrhoea, constipation and loss of appetite.

When the body is on high alert and prepared to fight or flee, then it might shut down functions that get in the way, such as digestion. We don't want to be wasting energy digesting our meal if we need that energy to escape or fight a tiger that wants to eat us. So, breathing and more passive poses will have a role in calming the nervous system so that we can take our body out of the high alert and dial more into our parasympathetic nervous system. This allows the body to start digesting again, and gives it a chance to repair, restore and nurture.

Exercises

Vinyasa for digestion

The simple daily sequence described in the 'Introduction' (page 12) can be very helpful in improving the flow of digestion, giving some space to the digestive organs. Try to get your breath to move down into your belly and digestive area (see Figures 7 to 11 on pages 22 to 25).

- Stretch your body fully as you **inhale**. Just take your arms as far as feels comfortable; you can interlace your fingers if needed, so you support an arm with a limited range of motion. One arm may go much further than the other arm. Be kind and compassionate to yourself and do not push through any pain.
- As you **exhale** hug your right knee into your chest. This is the **apanasana** –

71

the wind-relieving pose.
- **Inhale** stretching out and opening up the body.
- **Exhale** and hug your left knee into your chest.
- Continue… **inhale** stretching out, **exhale** hugging your right knee in, **inhale** stretching out, **exhale** hugging your left knee in.
- Then, next time you hug your right knee, circle the ankle around in one direction 3–4 times and then then the other direction 3–4 times. You can flex and point your foot and help to release the ankle joint.
- Then take your hands behind your right knee and, as you **inhale**, extend your right leg up towards the ceiling.
- **Exhale** and bend the leg.
- **Inhale** and extend the leg.
- If you feel these movements at all in your lower back, then you can bend your left knee and press your left foot into the floor.
- Repeat this 3–4 more times.

Figure-of-four

Next, work by adding on the **figure-of-four** pose.
- Cross your right ankle over, or on top of, your left knee. Pause for a moment and feel the space in your groin.
- This may be enough of a stretch for the gluteals (bottom muscles), but if you need to increase the stretch you can place a block under your left foot or draw your left knee in towards you.
- You can also interlace your fingers at the back of your left leg or use a strap to help lengthen your arms and hold the back of your leg instead.
- Try to soften your chest and shoulders. Notice if you transfer tension to your jaw, or your shoulders and neck.
- Breathe fully. Aim for an even count of your breath in and out.
- Repeat the sequence on the other side.

Supine twist

To finish the sequence, a **supine twist** can help to stimulate the function of the abdominal organs by alternately squeezing and then releasing. The idea with twists is that, when you release out of the twist, fresh oxygenated blood and nutrients rush into the organs and tissues.

- **Inhale**, draw your knees to the centre of your body and **exhale** twisting them halfway to the right.
- **Inhale** and pause (no movement).
- **Exhale** using your core to bring both knees up and over to the left.
- Repeat a few more times, moving on **exhale** so your core, and not your lower back, is supporting the movement (see Figure 21, page 48).
- You might like then to rest in the twist on each side for a few breaths, which gives space to one side and then the other of the digestive system.
- If you feel it in your lower back, then elevate the floor by putting cushions under or betwen your thighs so your knees stay hip-distance apart.
- Lengthen your top hip away from your face. Twists can be a big stretch into the chest area so you might want to change the angle of your arms so that you can open your chest and arms without any pain. You may experience a pulling sensation in your arm or armpit but should not be feeling any pain.

Supported child's pose

To finish, move into the **supported child's pose**. This is good for constipation but not diarrhoea as the shape of the pose allows us to soften and release any holding in the abdomen. This forward fold also brings our breath awareness into the back of the body.

This pose can be done over a bolster or with a pile of folded blankets instead: be generous with the towels or blankets as you may need them to support you in this pose (see Figure 36).

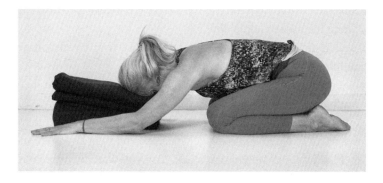

Figure 36: Supported child's pose

You can even draw the bolster or blankets in towards your body so it supports the front of your body and not just your head. If it is not comfortable to put pressure on your breasts or chest area, you can use blankets on top of your bolster to create space for your breasts so that there is no pain lying on the front of your body. You can be creative and use the props to mould around your body and elevate where you need a little lift. You might also need some blankets between your calves and hamstrings to give your knees a bit of space. If you feel that your hips are tight, then maybe make some more space beneath your pelvis and thighs by adding a blanket here or elevate the bolster by placing something underneath it.

Make sure you head is well supported and is on the bolster or blankets. Your chin and forehead should be level and even, with some support underneath your forehead. Turn your gaze to one side halfway through your restorative time and then change your gaze back to the other side in order to keep balance in your neck.

Allow your shoulder blades to soften down to the floor. You should feel gravity drawing them away from each other. Relax your arms and just settle and surrender and let any clenching or holding in your belly be released as you breathe. Breathe wide into the back of your body feeling your clothing being moved with your breath and as you exhale can you melt down into your support and feel how you are being held. You don't need to hold onto any tension. You can just release and let go.

Constipation

Breathing exercises can help the natural movement of the digestive system. The ascending colon is on the right side of the belly so waste travels up along the right side of the body, across the body on the transverse colon and then down the left side of the body along the descending colon.

- Start seated or lying down and begin to visualise your breath following this natural movement of the digestive system.
- As you breathe, sense breath travelling up the right side of your belly, across to the left and, as you **exhale**, down the left side of your body.
- As you follow your breath in this clockwise motion, observe if there are parts that are easier to breathe into or feel spacious and light and if are there areas that feel harder to breathe into or stuck. Can you direct your breathing to the 'stuck' areas as if your breath was a massage, massaging your body from the inside?

Diarrhoea

Supta baddha konasana

The supported **supta baddha konasana** can help to lift the diaphragm off the stomach and liver and can relieve indigestion, flatulence and/or diarrhoea.

- If you have a long belt or long scarf you can create a large loop in it.
- Place a bolster, or pile of folded towels or blankets, vertically a few inches behind you and sit in front of it with your knees bent.
- Place a folded blanket on the other end of the bolster for your head.
- Bend your knees to opposite sides and bring the soles of your feet together.
- Place the belt over your head and around your sacrum/pelvis.
- Pull the loop in front of you over your toes and underneath your feet so that the sides of the belt are on the inside edges of your legs.
- Now bring your feet closer to your pelvis and tighten the belt so that it is holding your legs close to your torso (see Figure 37).
- Don't make the belt so tight that you feel a pull on your knees.

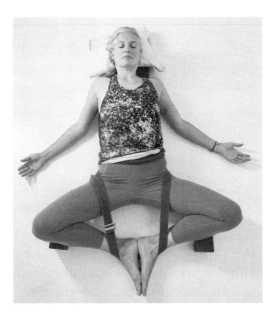

Figure 37: Supported supta baddha konasana

- Lie back over the bolster and place your head on the blanket so that your chin doesn't tilt back.
- With your hands, slide your sacrum and buttocks towards your feet so that your lower back feels long. If you feel any compression in your lower back, you may need to slide a bit more off the bolster towards your feet.
- Draw your shoulder blades away from your neck and roll the outer edges of your shoulders down so that your chest spreads from the centre to the sides. Let your arms release to your sides on the floor, spreading away from your chest, rotated outward, palms facing up.
- Place a cushion or yoga block underneath the outer edge of each leg. Close your eyes and rest for as long as you want to, up to 10 minutes (see Figure 38). Sense your breath moving down into your belly and allow your shoulder blades to feel as though they are sliding down the sides of the bolster and allowing gravity to open up your chest.
- Bring your awareness into your abdomen and breathe fully into your belly, allowing your belly to rise on inhale and fall on exhale.

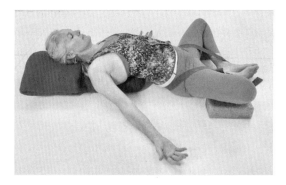

Figure 38: Resting in the supported supta baddha konasana

Supta baddha konasana is also a very important pose for prostate and bladder health. The blood circulates fully in the pelvis and abdomen. It is important that you use any props that you have to make yourself feel comfortable. Blankets (or towels), bolsters, cushions – anything that will reduce any tension in the pose so that you can rest deeply and heal. You can add on a massage to your belly, moving your hands in a clockwise direction for cramps and constipation and anticlockwise for diarrhoea.

Nausea and fatigue

The **Legs on chair** pose can help to reduce feelings of fatigue and nausea and stimulate movement of lymph fluid back down the legs towards the heart. Elevating the legs benefits the heart by increasing venous return, the amount of blood the heart receives which usually causes the heart to slow down and rest.

- You need to have two folded blankets, one for underneath your head and one that will go under your pelvis and lower back to keep your pelvis in neutral.
- Place a chair in front of you and sit on a folded blanket facing the chair. Take your legs over the chair so that your calves rest on the chair seat and lower yourself backwards onto the mat (see Figure 39).
- Adjust the blankets if needed so that your head is supported, there is space at your neck and your pelvis is in neutral.
- Breathe down into your belly. Can you sense your belly rise as you breathe in and fall as you breathe out?
- If you found the clockwise breathing following the anatomical path of your digestive system (page 74) useful, you could come back to breathing in and up the righthand side of your belly, across your belly and exhale down the lefthand side of your belly.
- You can stay in this pose for up to 20 minutes. Once you are ready to come out, roll to the side that is most comfortable for you; this may mean a stronger arm stays on top. Press down into the floor with your top hand and come up to sit. Your head will be the last thing to come up.

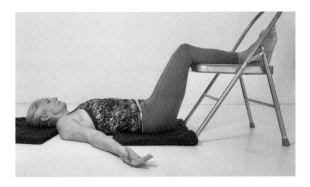

Figure 39: Legs on chair pose

Breathing techniques to calm the nervous system

There are breathing tools that are useful to help you stay with your breath and take some time in the present moment to calm your nervous system. Try one of the following to see if one works for you. They can be done lying down, seated or in one of the restorative poses.

- **Counting the breath**: Breathe in and then out for 3, 2, 1; breathe in for 3,2,1, breathe out for 4,3,2,1; breathe in for 4,3,2,1, breathe out for 5,4,3,2,1; breathe in for 5,4,3,2,1, and maybe stay with that count to see if you can lengthen your exhale so your breath out is a count longer than your inhale.
- **Opening your hands** as you breathe in and closing your hands into a gentle fist as you breathe out; repeat opening and closing your hands with your breathing.
- **Find a positive intention or affirmation** with your breath. Find two words that have meaning for you and support you today. For example, breathing in silently saying 'healthy' and as you breath out saying 'strong'. Breathing in 'calm' and breathing out 'centred'. What words resonate with you today?

You can stay in this pose for up to 20 minutes. If you are doing the pose lying down, once you are ready to come out roll to the side that is most comfortable for you; this may mean a stronger arm stays on top. Press down into the floor with your top hand and come up to sit. Your head will be the last thing to come up.

Mudras

The **apana vayu mudra** focuses on the subtle downward movement of energy in the body. It can be very grounding and cooling and good for the elimination of toxins and for constipation. Avoid practising it with diarrhoea.

- Bring your index finger to the base of your thumb. Bring your ring and middle fingers to touch the tip of the thumb and rest your hands on your lap (see Figure 27, page 61).
- Observe your breathing with the mudra. Is it easier to breathe? If it is harder to breathe then let go of the mudra. If not, explore how your breathing changes with the mudra. What happens if you let go of the mudra with one hand?

- Breathe in and breathe out. Does this change where you feel breath? Then change and let go of the mudra with your left hand. Observe any differences here.

According to yoga philosophy, **agni** or fire resides in the belly. This is our digestive strength, or power, and tradition says that if we stimulate this energy then we help the whole of the digestive system, allow our energy to flow more freely and can be more at ease in the body. When we breathe into our belly, we help to stoke this internal and digestive fire and, when we breathe out, we draw toxins into the fire to be eliminated or digested by it.

If you notice that your thoughts are not helpful to you today, you could also try visualising a fire in your belly and dropping those thoughts into the fire so you are fully digesting your experiences too. You could sense or see the colours red, orange and yellow. You could also try chanting **ram** (pronounced 'rum') and as you make the sound bring awareness down into your abdomen and lower back and visualise the sound waves massaging down into your digestive system and sense the vibrations of the sound stimulating the organs of your belly.

The **pushan mudra** in the chapter on 'Nausea' (page 168) can also be helpful for flatulence.

Everyday help for digestion

Posture can also restrict our digestion. If we round our spine when we are sitting, and our chest closes and our shoulders round, the blood flow gets restricted and the colon gets a little squashed (see Figure 40). If we aren't breathing fully or our diaphragm is constricted, then our internal organs can't get nourished and massaged by the movement of our diaphragm. So, creating length in our spine and breathing into our belly will help with digestion by increasing blood flow and internal movement to the digestive system.

Find the natural curves when you are seated. Check you are sitting on your sitting bones and not rounding back onto your tailbone. Sense that your lower back is moving forward rather than rounding back behind you (see Figure 41).

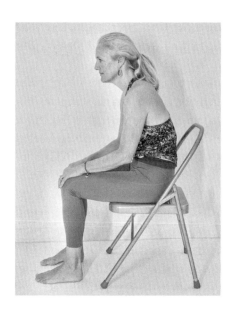

Figure 40: Slumped position that does not aid digestion

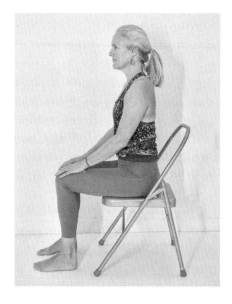

Figure 41: Posture that helps digestion

Eyes – dry, watery and itchy

Dry or watery eyes are not such commonly known side effects of cancer treatment but can be a constant reminder of living with cancer. Simple yoga exercises can help rejuvenate the eyes by resting over-used muscles, reducing tension in the face and eyes and strengthening muscles that help the eyes focus.

Rub your hands together for 10 to 15 seconds until they feel warm and energised. Then cup them and gently place them over your eyes, with your fingertips resting on your forehead. Close your eyes, breathe deeply and relax. Feel the warmth and energy from your hands and allow your eyes to grow soft and spacious and to enjoy this break from visual stimulation.

- Visualise a clock face.
- Look up at 12 and down at 6. Look from 6 to 12 then over to 3 and across to 9. Look from 9 to 3.
- Then follow this sequence: look up at 12 and down to 6, up to 1 and down to 7, up to 2 and down to 8, across to 3 and across to 9, down to 4 and up to 10, down to 5 and up to 11, then down to 6 and up to 12.
- Then back: 7 and 1, 8 and 2, 9 and 3, 10 and 4, 11 and 5, 12 and then 6.
- Close your eyes for a moment.
- Then circle your eyes – follow your eyes around a clock face from 12 back to 12 in a clockwise direction three times and then change direction and go anticlockwise three times.

We are bombarded by images all the time; this can be completely exhausting for our senses, and we can get a feeling of sensory overload. When our energy, or prana, is constantly moving outwards, we can get overwhelmed and exhausted and feel that our energy is being drained away.

If we can shift our attention and energy away from the external world, we can find we actually refresh a little. Taking time to just sit with our eyes closed when waiting for appointments or travelling on public transport can give us a little break and I find, when relaxing in savasana, that placing something over my eyes, like an eye pillow, helps to shut out the light and really helps me to relax.

Fatigue

Hendersen reports that cancer-related fatigue (CRF) is one of the most frequently reported side effects among those impacted by cancer.[1] She describes it as 'a persistent sense of exhaustion that is not alleviated by sleep or rest and that interferes significantly with the person's usual functioning'. Hendersen reports on research carried out by the German Cancer Research Centre (DKFZ), which 'initially evaluated the patterns, severity and management of CRF among 2,508 patients with 15 different types of cancer two years after the discovery of their illness'. She then notes that 'in a follow-up survey… almost 40% of survivors continued to report fatigue that they rated as a moderate or severe burden. In addition to fatigue, more than 40% of patients reported being at least moderately burdened by loss of physical capacity and over one third suffered from trouble sleeping, sexual problems, joint pains and anxiety'.

So, CRF can be a huge issue for many people. This may also be combined with insomnia, and you can feel 'tired and wired', where you feel physically tired but your mind is really busy, making it hard to relax and go to sleep.

Fatigue can also be due to the loss of muscle mass that we experience when we are more sedentary. Periods of time in hospital, of bed rest or of being unable to exercise, lead to losing muscle mass. This means that normal everyday activities are harder to do as we don't have as much strength. So, although it sounds counterintuitive to exercise when feeling exhausted, if you can follow some of the sequences in the 'Weakness in muscles – building strength' (page 247) and 'Osteoporosis' (page 171) chapters, then these will help you keep muscle mass and therefore not be as exhausted moving about your daily activities.

Research shows that yoga interventions can improve sleep and reduce persistent fatigue. All this can help to boost quality of life, as we often feel we can cope with things better when we have had a good night's sleep. In a randomised controlled trial of breast cancer survivors, participants who practised a twice-weekly 90-minute hatha class for 12 weeks reported less fatigue and more vitality. They also showed a decrease in inflammation.[2]

The following poses are restorative and designed to soothe the nervous system without being depleting. When we are fatigued, we often round our shoulders and our chest and diaphragm (our main breathing muscle) get compressed; it can't then move through its full range of motion, and this makes it more challenging to breathe fully. When we open up our chest, we feel more energised. You can explore this yourself right now by noticing how you feel if you allow your body to slump, shoulders to round and head to drop. Then change and sit up tall, roll your shoulders back and open your chest and notice if this feels better?

The props used in restorative yoga should fully support the body and allow you to open up the front of your body so your chest can expand without too much physical effort and the practice is not draining you of energy. As you are held by all the props, you can just release and let go into the supported pose. Let gravity and the supports do the work.

Restorative poses

Supta baddha konasana

This pose has already been described in the chapters on 'Colostomy, ostomy, ileostomy and yoga with a stoma' (page 59) and 'Digestive problems and discomfort' (page 71), but it is also valuable for addressing fatigue.

- If you have a belt or long scarf, you can create a large loop in your belt.
- Place a bolster or a pile of folded towels or blankets vertically a few inches behind you and sit in front of it with your knees bent. Have a folded blanket on the other end of the bolster for your head.
- Bend your knees to the sides and bring the soles of your feet together. Place the belt over your head and around your sacrum/pelvis. Pull the loop in front of you over your toes and underneath your feet so that the sides of the belt are on the inside edges of your legs (see Figure 37, page 75).
- Now bring your feet closer to your pelvis and tighten the belt so that it is holding your legs close to your torso. Don't make the belt so tight that you

feel a pull on your knees.
- Lie back over the bolster and place your head on the blanket so that your chin doesn't tilt back. With your hands slide your sacrum and buttocks toward your feet so that your lower back feels long. If you feel any compression in the lower back, you may need to slide a bit more off the bolster toward your feet.
- Pull your shoulder blades away from your neck and roll the outer edges of your shoulders down so that your chest spreads from the centre to the sides. Let your arms release to your sides on the floor, spreading away from your chest, rotated outward, palms facing up.
- Place a cushion or yoga block underneath the outer edge of each leg. Close your eyes and rest for up to 10 minutes. Sense your breath moving down into your belly and allow your shoulder blades to feel like they are sliding down the sides of the bolster and allowing gravity to open up your chest (see Figure 38, page 76).

Viparita karani with blankets

This pose is calming for the nervous system and is also known as 'Legs up the wall'. It turns the body upside down to give it a break from its normal functioning of having to pump blood back towards the heart. It also increases the blood flow to the pelvis and abdomen, which can be beneficial for digestive distress as well.
- Place a folded blanket near a wall.
- Sit with your right outer hip on the blanket so your sitting bones are touching the wall.
- Use your hands behind you on the floor to support you as you roll your sacrum onto the blanket and your legs up the wall.
- Push your hands into the floor to push your hips closer to the wall.
- Gently lower your head and shoulders to the floor, keeping your hips close to the wall so that your legs don't lean but are supported and you feel your thighbones descending down into your pelvis.
- Stay in this position for up to 15 minutes (see Figure 42).

To come out of the pose:
- Bend your knees and roll to one side. If you feel like you don't have enough space, then press your feet into the wall to push yourself away from it so you can roll to the side that is most comfortable to you and come up.

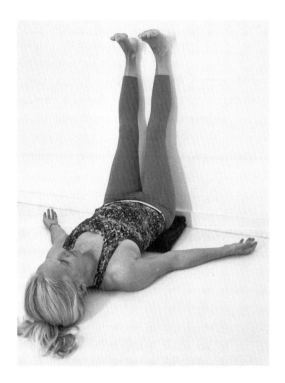

Figure 42: Viparita karani with blankets

Mudras for fatigue

You could also try a mudra.

Starting seated or lying down, bring your awareness to your breathing and notice where you are feeling your breath. Can you breathe down into your belly or is your breath getting stuck somewhere?

Observe a few rounds of breathing to see if you can start to direct your breath into the areas of your body that are not receiving it. Then try making a **prana mudra** – that is, a mudra to help encourage the prana or energy into your body. Gertrud Hirschi says in *Mudras – Yoga in Your Hands* that prana mudra 'generally increases vitality, reduces fatigue and nervousness and improves vison'.[3] Bring the thumb, little and ring fingers to touch on both hands (see Figure 43).

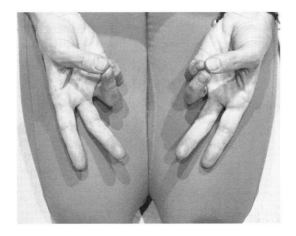

Figure 43: The prana mudra

Whilst holding your hands in the prana mudra, rest the back of your hands on the floor if you are lying down or rest them on your lap if you are seated. Now notice if this changes where you are feeling your breath. Is it easier to breathe and get breath into your body? If you have a negative reaction – it becomes harder to breathe or you feel lightheaded or nauseous – then release the mudra.

Breathing techniques for fatigue

You can incorporate little exercises throughout your day to keep your muscles strong. See daily suggestions in the chapter on 'Weakness in muscles – building strength' (page xx). But so often when we are exhausted, we don't feel like doing anything. As we will explore in that chapter, the less we move the harder it is to move and the more we move and get our muscles working, the easier it will be to move and therefore it will be less exhausting. So, what can we do to energise ourselves to be motivated to get up and onto our mats to stretch and strengthen our fabulous bodies?

Yoga has some breathing techniques that are said to be energising. We will look at alternate nostril breathing for balance (page 88) and also to help us calm to go to sleep (page 267), but we can use the same technique of breathing through our right nostril to stimulate the brain and energise us. This technique is known as **surya bhedana**. 'Surya' is Sanskrit for the sun.

Surya bhedana

Traditionally you would first bring your hands into a **vishnu mudra** (also known as **mrigi mudra**), where the index and middle finger are placed on the base of the thumb, leaving the ring finger and the thumb to close off the nostrils.

- Close your left nostril just where you feel your nose goes from bone to cartilage and not at the bottom of the nostrils where they can get stuck closed. If the nostrils get stuck it can make your gasp for air and create a sense of stress which is the opposite of what we are trying to achieve.
- Close your left nostril very gently with your ring finger and thumb.
- **Inhale** through your **right** nostril and then close it at the top of the inhale and exhale out through your **left** nostril.
- Close your **left** nostril at the end of the exhale and then **inhale** through your **right** nostril; then close your **right** nostril and **exhale** out through the **left**.
- Continue this (inhaling through the right nostril and exhaling through the left) for 1–3 minutes.

Viloma 1

Another breathing exercise, **viloma 1** can also help to energise the body as it focuses on the inhale. Our inhales are energising and stimulate the sympathetic side of our autonomic nervous system (see page 35).

- Find a comfortable seated position where your spine feels long and you don't feel like you are slumping into your lower back. You could be sitting on a chair, or on the floor on a cushion or blanket.
- Take a breath in through your nose and a breath out through your mouth.
- Then if you are not congested, continue to breathe in and out through your nose. Can you feel your breath moving down into your belly? Sense your body expanding as you inhale and softening and letting go as you exhale.
- On your next **inhale**, breathe in **halfway** and pause.
- Then **breathe in fully**, pause at the top of your inhale and, keeping the length and height you have created, **breathe out fully**.
- Repeat 2–3 more times.

If this feels comfortable, you can start to breathe in in thirds.
- **Breathe in a third**, then pause.
- **Breathe in a second third**, then pause again.
- **Breathe in fully** all the way to the top and pause.
- **Exhale fully** all your breath out.
- Repeat 2–3 more times.

You could then add on moving your arms with your breathing. I find that by elevating my arms, I feel like I can breathe a little more deeply.
- Start with your arms down by your side and turn your palms forward.
- **Inhale** a third and float your arms out a third to the side.
- **Inhale** a second third and float your arms a little higher.
- **Inhale** fully, floating your arms to the sky.
- Pause, then **exhale** fully all your breath out.
- Repeat 2–3 more times.
- Then pause and notice the effects on your breathing.

Energising movements

Explore whether some small movements can also be energising. Lying on your back, take your legs and arms up to the ceiling and give everything a good shake (see Figure 44), as though you were shaking the muscle away from the bone.

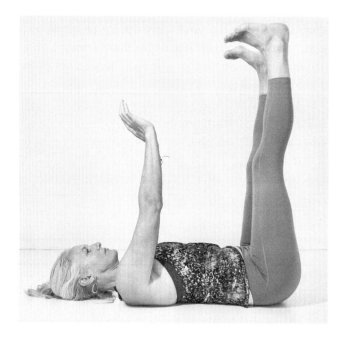

Figure 44: Shaking arms and legs

When you are finished, come into **savasana** (the rest pose – see page xx) and feel your body tingling or being stimulated.

If you now feel a little more energised you could try moving through the warm-up sequence in the Introduction (see Figures 1 to 16, pages 19–29).

Grief

Grief is a response to the loss of something. A person, a part of your body or the life you were having before you were diagnosed with cancer. Loss of 'normal life', whatever that might be, or the loss of what we thought we knew or of what could have been. It is completely normal that, when you start to practise yoga and become in tune with your changing body, you can be overwhelmed with a sense of grief and loss. The emotional pain that you can experience in your heart and mind (emotionally and mentally) can feel just as strong and powerful as physical pain and often in my classes people are moved to tears as everything they have gone through or are going through comes bubbling to the surface.

How can we live with this loss? There is no right or wrong way to grieve; your feelings are *your feelings* and it is important to let them come to the surface and to be able to hear and validate what you are experiencing in this moment. Your feelings are not 'good' or 'bad' or 'right' or 'wrong', or any other label that you might attach to them. Can you instead observe all that you are feeling with a non-judgemental mind? Be kind to these thoughts as you would be to a small child who was upset and grieving, and simply feel fully what you are feeling right now without adding more thoughts in the form of labels and judgements.

The thing about grief is, because it is painful and we don't like pain, we try to avoid feeling it. This may also be exacerbated by lack of sleep and/or physical pain, and we react because we just don't know what to do. We busy and distract ourselves and try to push away these uncomfortable and often all-consuming, overwhelming feelings. Sometimes this is just the only way we can deal with something in this moment in time. It's just too painful to cope with on top of everything else we are coping with. So, we shove things back down away from the surface so that we can get on with the things that are our priority right now.

However, if you hold a beach ball under the water, the further you push it down the higher it will jump. At some point we need to acknowledge in the first person that 'I am grieving,' … 'I am deeply sad and feeling the loss of…'. Start to observe what you are feeling and where in your body you might be feeling grief and don't ignore it or push it away. The physical practices in this book help us to release tension and bring awareness to what is happening in our physical body. Moving with our breathing, brings us back again and again to our breath and that disrupts our habit of ruminating when our ruminations can be haunting, scary and more frightening than our reality. Can you be kind to whatever thoughts come up so that you start to befriend your experiences, even the ones you don't like?

By not avoiding pain and instead acknowledging and feeling it, we take the edge off it. By not suppressing these emotions or feelings we don't allow them to completely preoccupy us and get stuck in our bodies. We want to feel fully and then release fully. If we can be fully present with feelings of grief, knowing what we are feeling and feeling it fully, then this is the start of the healing process. By engaging with these painful feelings we are less likely to identify with being a victim of our emotions and feelings because by living through grief and recognising it is happening inside of us we do actually take back some control. It is not completely outside of our control anymore as whilst we become present with these emotions we can possibly start to relate to them and nurture them rather than feeling a victim to them. This is what makes us, as human beings, incredibly resilient. Just think about what you have already endured in your life and the different strategies you may have used to cope with the shock or trauma of being diagnosed with cancer and how you may have already found ways to create conditions in your life to help repair from the traumatic effect of diagnosis.

We have this innate strength and wisdom deep inside of us which I see regularly in the classes I teach. It is this wisdom that can help us when we observe that we are not our thoughts, our feelings or our mind. We have a mind and our mind has feelings and thoughts but these are also not completely accurate. The voice inside our head sounds like us so it is very believable but is not always a reliable source and can often be unhelpful in the repairing process. The chapter on Referred pain (page 201) explores the concept of primary and secondary pain further, but primary pain is the actual feeling of pain and secondary pain relates to the thoughts we attach to those sensations and the stories we tell ourselves about that pain.

We do need time to listen to what is going on inside, even though this can be hugely painful, and we need to recognise this without any judgement but also to be able to observe when our mind is creating a narrative that is not accurate or helpful and preventing us moving on. However, there is no right or wrong way to grieve.

Sometimes you might just want to be left alone to deal with your life at your own pace and other times through this grief you may be open to receiving love and encouragement from friends and family, or find the strength and support from your wider cancer community. This might be through social media or through charities. Instagram has a wonderful cancer community that shares and supports each other and maybe reading others accounts may help you feel less alone or give your some guidance on what to do. Maybe you need some professional external support; Macmillan provide a cancer support line (0808 808 0000) and run a telephone buddy scheme to ensure that you feel supported and are not facing cancer alone. It may be that you find things or people in life that give life meaning because when we have meaning we also have hope.

With support we might find that it is possible to befriend all these challenging emotions because it is a process. It is a process and a practice that are always 'work in progress' to cultivate kindness towards all our feelings – the good, the bad and the ugly.

The irony is that it takes stopping and pausing and taking time to *be* a human being, and not a human *doing*, to start to be fully aware of what we are actually feeling in this moment. This is why yoga can feel so challenging as you roll out your yoga mat, turn off your phone and your other distractions and stop. In this quieting down we can suddenly be aware of how we are actually feeling, physically and mentally. In this stillness we can see how many thoughts we are having and if those thoughts are focusing on the past or the future. Are we going over things that have happened or things that haven't happened? Or are those thoughts just going round and round on a loop? Sometimes our yoga mat can be the most painful place to be, and it is easy to feel frustrated, sad or angry and want to get off our mat and go back to being distracted by life.

However, if we can try to add a cultivation of kindness, a befriending of all these different complex feelings, it has the potential to be freeing. It allows you to be with whatever it is that you find directly under your nose and be more awake to life. By being really present and fully conscious we stop being on autopilot and sleepwalking through our life. We get the opportunity to engage with the fullness of this rollercoaster of life – its ups and downs – and this can be empowering; challenging, but powerful.

Yoga techniques to try

Three-part breathing

When we are stressed or anxious, we often hold our breath; this triggers alarms which tell our body something is wrong. So maybe we can use our breathing to defuse any suffering or distress? Try the three-part breathing in the chapter on 'Breathing' (see page 43). See if this whole-body breathing which stimulates the calming parasympathetic system can help to release tension and start to create feelings of peace or serenity as an antidote to pain.

Mukula mudra

To conclude this chapter, this simple and easy-to-do mudra helps you to breathe into your heart. You bring the fingers of one hand to touch their respective thumb and repeat the same with the opposite hand. The hands now look a little bit like bird beaks (see Figure 45).

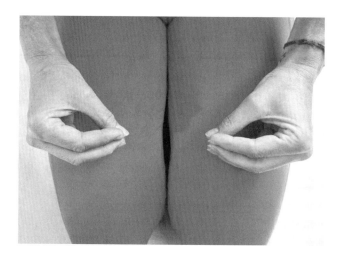

Figure 45: The mukula mudra

Now focus your awareness on your heart. Can you breathe into your heart as if there was a camera lens there that opened to allow you to breathe directly into your heart and sense how your heart expands when you focus your breath there? It can feel more vibrant as it fills with vital energy.

After a few rounds of breathing into your heart, start to send that breath down into your hands and fingers.

Then, placing your hands on an area of your body that needs more love, sense breath and love from your heart moving down to your hands and into the area of your body that you want to benefit from this love.

Begin slowly with a few breaths and then build up to 5 minutes with the mudra. Observe what it feels like.

As with all mudras, if this makes you feel lightheaded or nauseous or it makes it harder to breathe, then let go of this mudra.

The loving kindness meditation in the chapter on the 'Immune system and infections' (page 104) can also be supportive in dealing with feelings of grief.

Hot flushes

The drop in oestrogen caused by some medications or surgery can create changes in the body that may include hot flushes. This chapter focuses on practices which are energetically more calming for the body as hot flushes can reoccur when stressed. You can experiment with some of the poses in this book to find what works for you to make your feel calmer and reduce the sensation of hot flushes.

In *Relax and Renew: Restful Yoga for Stressful Times*, Judith Hanson Lasater describes hot flushes as the energy or prana moving from the centre of the body outwards towards the periphery, heating your skin.[1] She says that inversion draws the prana inwards towards your organs and away from the skin surfaces. This helps to cool the body back down. So, a good practice is the restorative pose 'Legs up the wall', also known as **viparita karani**.

Restorative poses

Viparita karani with blankets

This pose is calming for the nervous system. It turns the body upside down, so it gives it a break from its normal function of having to pump blood back upwards towards the heart. It also increases blood flow to the pelvis.

- Place two folded blankets next to a wall.
- Sit with your right outer hip on the blankets so you are close to the wall. If your right side is tender you may prefer to sit with your left hip close to the wall so the next steps are more comfortable. Use your hands behind you on the floor to support you as you roll your sacrum onto the blanket and your

legs up the wall. Push your hands into the floor to push your hips closer to the wall.

- Gently lower your head and shoulders to the floor, keeping your hips close to the wall so that your legs don't lean but are supported and you feel your thighbones descending down into your pelvis (see Figure 42, page 86).
- Stay in this position for 5–15 minutes. You can also move your legs wide into a V-shape if that is comfortable for you (see Figure 46).
- You can also use a strap and create a loop about hip distance apart and loop it around your shins, so your legs are held as they relax. They can press out into the strap and be supported.

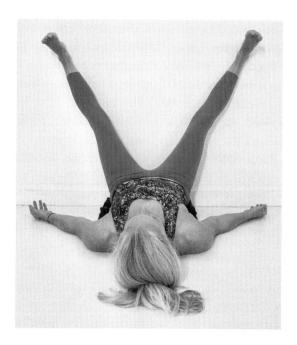

Figure 46: Legs up the wall in V-shape position

Supta baddha konasana

This is another pose which is helpful for hot flushes.
- If you have a belt or long scarf, create a large loop.
- Place a bolster or a pile of folded towels or blankets vertically a few inches

behind you and sit in front of it with your knees bent.

- Have a folded blanket on the other end of the bolster for your head.
- Bend your knees to the sides and bring the soles of your feet together.
- Place the belt or scarf around your sacrum/pelvis like a belt, making sure it isn't around your lower back.
- Pull the loop in front of you on the inside of your legs and bring the under sides of your feet into the loop. The strap will then hold your feet in place to stop them sliding away from your body. This should allow your legs to relax fully.
- Now bring your feet closer to your pelvis and tighten the belt or scarf so that it is holding your legs close to your torso. Don't make it so tight that you feel a pull on your knees.
- Lie back over the bolster and place your head on the blanket so that your chin doesn't tilt back.
- With your hands, slide your sacrum and buttocks towards your feet so that your lower back feels long. If you feel any compression in your lower back, you may need to slide a bit more off the bolster towards your feet (see Figure 38, page 76).
- Pull your shoulder blades away from your neck and roll the outer edges of your shoulders down so that your chest spreads from the centre to the sides. Let your arms release to your sides on the floor, spreading away from your chest, rotated outward, palms facing up.
- Place a cushion or yoga block underneath the outer edge of each leg. Close your eyes and rest for up to 10 minutes. Sense your breath moving down into your belly and allow your shoulder blades to feel as though they are sliding down the sides of the bolster and allowing gravity to open up your chest.

Cooling breathing techniques

Sitali

Cooling breathing techniques, such as **sitali** or **sikali**, can help you calm and have a sense of taking back some control, which may help with the frequency of hot flushes and make you feel less stressed by them.

The ability to curl your tongue is genetically determined; curl it for this technique if you can, but if you can't, you can make a circle with your mouth and breathe in like breathing in through a straw, or you can suck air in through the sides of your teeth.

- Start to feel the cool air firstly in your mouth and throat.
- Breathe out through your nose. Visualise warmth from inside your body releasing out through your nose.
- As you continue you can visualise or feel the cool air travelling down into your chest, sense your chest cooling and, as you breathe out, feel warmth from inside your chest coming out with your exhale through your nose.
- Breathe in through your nose and feel cool air travelling down into your abdomen; then exhale any heat and warmth out through your nose with your exhale.
- Inhale sending cool breath down into your pelvis and then as you breathe out, send the heat from your pelvis out through your nose.
- You can stay with this breathing pattern for a few minutes and observe any cooling sensations in your body.

When we stimulate the tongue whilst breathing like this, we can also help to bring a vibration or massaging affect to the vagus nerve. The vagus nerve is a long cranial nerve with many branches that wanders through the body from the brain stem into the chest and abdomen to regulate many of the visceral organs. It supplies nerves to the respiratory system, the digestive system, the circulatory system and the organs of elimination (kidneys) and is part of the parasympathetic nervous system. It helps to calm us and trigger a relaxation response in the body.

Deep breathing or focusing on our breathing is one way we can stimulate the healthy functioning of the vagus nerve. Singing or humming is another way to stimulate the vagus nerve.

Immune system and infections

The immune system is our defence against all things foreign. Our individual immune systems are all different and, like our fingerprints, unique to us.

The immune system is active everywhere in the body and is always on the look out for invaders and unhealthy cells and ready to respond to attack by creating an immune response. It consists of a network of cells, tissues and organs which work as a whole to protect us; these permeate every system in the body. The respiratory, skin, musculoskeletal, nervous, endocrine, lymphatic and digestive systems all work together as a team to fight against infection and illness. For example, salivary glands inside our mouth protect us from the microbes that we are exposed to in our food, drink and the air we breathe. Cells in these glands produce an antibody called immunoglobulin A (IgA), which are our first line of defence. Alongside antibodies, the immune system produces T-cells that are the powerhouse of the immune response and are a type of white blood cell. They are made in the spongy tissue inside our bones called bone marrow. T-cell function is regulated by another type of white blood cell – neutrophils.

Certain treatments for cancer affect our immune system because they are designed to attack fast-growing cancer cells in the body but also attack other fast-growing cells including those in the bone marrow; this reduces the number of white blood cells. Chemo can cause neutropenia (a decrease in the number of neutrophils). This can reduce the body's ability to fight infection and might show up as a fever, chills or sweating. Even immunotherapy that helps the body have a better reaction against cancer cells can change the way the immune system works and can also lead to an increased risk of infection due to a weakening of the immune system.

Our bone marrow also produces the red blood cells that carry oxygen and the platelets that help our blood to clot. A low red blood cell count can lead to fatigue, chest pain, dizziness and being short of breath.

Yoga stimulates the musculoskeletal system by strengthening muscles and bones; these muscles in turn stimulate the lymphatic system, another crucial part of the immune system that is responsible for draining and filtering out toxins, dead cells and other waste matter from around the body. It flows in one direction from the periphery (the farthest parts of the body) back towards the heart and into the bloodstream, and relies on muscle movement to work optimally. It is worth noting for any days when you might feel too exhausted to move physically that even by breathing fully and diaphragmatically we also help the movement of fluids (lymph and blood) back towards our heart by stimulating the thoracic duct (the largest lymphatic vessel in the body) and that breathing fully therefore stimulates the immune system.

When we are breathing fully, we are also helping our cells receive energy through our breath and we can survive for periods of time without food or water but we can't survive without breathing. Our breath literally gives us life, and we can visualise that, as we breathe in, we are drawing energy and life into our bodies to support and strengthen us.

It is widely recognised now that our immune system is also in our gut, with an estimated 70–80% of all immune cells being located there.[1, 2, 3] We know that when we calm our body, we stimulate the 'rest and digest' response, helping the functioning of the digestive system. So, any of the chapters in this book will help to support the immune system.

Kindness strengthens immunity

Chronic stress suppresses the immune system due to the release of cortisol, a hormone that activates the sympathetic nervous system. Cortisol, a steroid hormone, reduces inflammation and inflammation is an essential part of the immune response. (It is thought that cortisol reduces inflammation to protect the immune system and stop it becoming overactive to facilitate the fight or flight response which would be weakened by inflammation.) Cortisol increases bone resorption (the break down of bone by creating osteoclast cells) and, when it is chronically elevated, can affect bone density. Restorative practices that help to soothe the nervous system will help to reduce feelings of stress and therefore the production of cortisol.[4] See the chapters on

'Nausea' (page 165) and 'Fatigue' (page 83) for restorative postures and the chapter on 'Osteoporosis' (page 171) for building bone strength.

When we are anxious and feel like life is out of our control, we experience emotions that are central to the experience of stress and our immune system is less effective when we are in conflict. There are studies that show that positive emotions promote and foster a stronger immune system. Researchers at Harvard University carried out a study where participants watched videos of Mother Theresa carrying out acts of kindness and compassion and found that simply observing these acts boosted the participants' immune system; this was named the 'Mother Theresa effect'.[5] It was measured by an increase in IgA in participants' saliva (the immune system's first line of defence against invaders, as explained above). Participants' perception of goodness and kindness, even though it was just observing someone else being kind, helped increase their immune function. It has also been found that premature babies who are shown love gain weight faster and get to leave hospital sooner.[6]

The impact that love, connection and kindness can have on our health was also highlighted in 1978 when an experiment to look at the relationship between high blood cholesterol and heart health discovered that kind treatment of the rabbits being studied helped them to become healthier. This research by Dr Robert Nerem was documented in *The Rabbit Effect* by Kelli Harding.[7] The researchers found that for some of the lab rabbits being nurtured and stroked by a kind researcher as they were fed their high cholesterol diet made the difference between them having a heart attack and a healthy heart. The rabbits that were loved had 60% less plaque in their arteries than the rabbits that were ignored, even though they were on the same diet.

David Hamilton has written many books on the power of kindness to affect your health, and he writes in *The Five Side Effects of Kindness* that 'kindness can diffuse stress and the things that trigger it …worry anxiety and fear'.[8] Our brains are highly plastic and constantly adapting. The prefrontal cortex builds like a muscle when we meditate. Our brain can't tell the difference between us actually doing something and imagining doing it. If we behave in a kind way or we recall acts of kindness or even watch videos of kindness, as with the Mother Theresa study, we release oxytocin which has an effect on our heart. Oxytocin is a cardio-protective hormone as it allows tension in the walls of arteries to release and more blood to reach the heart, leading to a decrease in blood pressure. So, observe what you are feeding your heart in terms of what you tell yourself. We are our worst critics and can be really unkind to ourselves when we would never consider saying the same things to another person. Can you allow yourself a little smile when you notice your mind wandering so you develop an attitude of gentleness and kindness towards your thoughts?

We also release oxytocin, a happy hormone, when we are hugged, touched or have feelings of love, and oxytocin slows down the growth and spread of both breast and ovarian cancers.[9] Feelings of love create a sense of being safe, belonging and that the body can start to begin to repair.[10] Certain areas of the body have receptor sites for oxytocin which means that they are highly responsive to oxytocin's healing effects, which all helps to stimulate the immune system.[11]

Studies show that kindness also helps to lower inflammation.[12] Inflammation is a natural immune response and is the body drawing blood and nutrients to an area that is under attack but if it is not resolved, then prolonged or chronic inflammation can lead to a number of serious health problems. Loving kindness, or metta, also helps to defuse chronic pain and suffering and boosts positive emotions.[13]

Metta = kindness to reduce inflammation and boost oxytocin

The Buddhist tradition has a meditation called a **metta meditation**, meaning positive energy and kindness. It helps to create loving kindness for all beings, including ourselves. If we can develop kindness and compassion towards what is happening in our lives, then we can be part of and present in this challenging life without being reactive. And if we can create enough loving kindness for ourselves then maybe we can start to pass this on to others.

Patanjali explores this in Sutra 1.33 when he guides us to cultivate an attitude of friendship towards those who are happy, of compassion to those who are suffering, of joy to those who are virtuous and of equanimity towards those who are not virtuous, so we don't feel division or hatred.[14] The sutra states that if we cultivate these feelings then the 'mind stuff retains its undisturbed calmness'.

In challenging times, it can be really hard to celebrate other peoples' happiness as it may bring up feelings of envy or jealousy. We can end up focusing on what we lack or why we are going through something, but if we can celebrate goodness in others then it helps to bring forward our own goodness which cultivates an inner attitude of compassion for everyone, including ourselves. We aren't getting pulled off centre by our thoughts or getting caught up in other people's or reacting to others, which can just increase our sense of suffering or create a sense of isolation. The Buddhist tradition suggests that you should:

Breathe in kindliness and acceptance towards all that you experience.
Breathe out kindliness and tenderness to all that you experience.

This meditation creates a wish that someone is not suffering and not in any pain and that they might sense or start to nurture feelings of love. It is easy to wish well to the people you love, but it is harder to do so to the people that you don't like, and even harder to wish well to those that you know cause suffering to others. However, if we can send kindness to those people then maybe they will find more happiness, suffer less and mistreat others less.

Meditations

We can use affirmations – positive words that we repeat to ourselves. Here are some suggestions:
- May I be patient and strong.
- May I be free from fear and pain.
- May I be contented with the way things are.
- May I be happy and healthy.
- May I know peace in the world.
- May I be free from suffering.
- May my body be filled with healing energy.

Find words that resonate with *you* and that have meaning to *you*. Say them out loud. Say them to yourself. What would you wish for? What supports you right now? After each phrase take a deep breath and notice how it feels in your body.

This practice could be done in a seated position or lying over a bolster in a heart-opening pose like supta baddha konasana (see page 75).
- Bring your awareness to your breathing. Feel your breath in your abdomen, maybe even placing hands on your belly or one hand on your heart and another on your belly. See if you can be in a place of observation.
- Be aware of the thoughts that come up. Notice what is arising but don't fight your thoughts; accept or be at peace with what comes up. Use your breathing to anchor you into this moment.
- Steady your breathing and be aware of all the sounds around you without being caught up in what you are hearing and your thoughts about them.

- Be aware of the sensations that arise without getting caught up in what those sensations might mean, whether they are pleasant, unpleasant or neutral. Even if we notice discomfort can we just notice that discomfort is discomfort without adding any reactions? Don't lean towards or pull away from any sensations. Be curious. Observe. Just be aware with no reaction.
- Feel with each breath your body becoming more at ease.

Bring your awareness to your heart. Sense your physical (anatomical) heart and then sense your emotional or energetic heart centre. The heart is the centre of love and compassion but also strength. Can you imagine breathing into your heart and feeling it fill with breath and vital energy? Sense your heart becoming full and vibrant. Then, starting with yourself, notice that it can be challenging to be loving to yourself, but what if you viewed yourself as if you were a child? Is it easier to be loving to a five-year-old version of yourself? Recall the feeling of being with someone you love. Feel this love deeply. Sense it moving through your heart. How does it feel to generate love for someone you love? Is that an easier place to start? How does it feel? What sensations do you observe? What parts of your body respond to this feeling? Then say to yourself either the words that you are working with or possibly these suggestions:

- May I be happy.
- May I be healthy.
- May I be full of loving kindness.

You might even sense golden or white light in your heart as you say the words, stimulating a feeling of metta towards yourself.

Sense this love flowing from your heart now out to a friend or person you care for. Picture them, seeing them and their qualities in your mind's eye, maybe repeating your words directed to them. Visualise sending light from your heart to theirs, maybe allowing it to flow out from your heart with your breath to more people you know well or care for.

Then can you extend loving kindness out to someone you do not know very well or for whom your feelings are neutral (neither disliking or liking them). Take a moment to reflect on them. We often overlook 'neutral' people – people we have no opinions about but can make instant decisions about based on very little data. Send them wishes that they suffer less; that they might be truly happy, maybe repeating the words that resonated with you. Visualise sending light from your heart to theirs.

Now sense the feeling extending out of your immediate world to reach out to include someone you dislike or find difficult to get on with. Without analysing your choice, observe the feelings that come up when you think about this person but do not get caught up in feelings of hate. This is the most challenging because it puts us out of our comfort zone. It doesn't make their behaviour acceptable or mean we condone it, but it does recognise that we are all human and we all react sometimes because we are in pain, or we are suffering. Many factors can make people become challenging or difficult. As you reflect on them maybe you can visualise them as a small child or vulnerable as a way of being able to offer out loving kindness to them. Repeat your chosen phrases.

Visualise sending light from your heart to theirs. No one is immune to suffering so sense that their behaviour may be due to their struggles. Send your metta to them as well. This may not feel very genuine at first but notice how it feels and know that, by repetition and practice, it will start to feel more real and less fake.

Allow loving kindness to flow out to people you know exist, but you don't know them personally; sense this growing bigger and bigger until it starts to become universal. Can you send loving kindness to someone who is in pain, someone who is caring for someone who is sick, someone who is worried? Sense that wave of loving kindness spreading out beyond into the world. To all beings everywhere.

Gratitude

Finding gratitude when you have been diagnosed with cancer might just be one of the hardest things to do, but evidence shows that a daily gratitude practice can help boost immunity. A recent study at the University of California San Diego's school of medicine found that people who had a gratitude practice had better heart health, specifically less inflammation.[15] Studies also show that practices of gratitude reduce stress, depression and anxiety and increase wellbeing.[16] A practice of gratitude connects us to something. That might be a small flower, a person, a thing, or a situation. Connection stops us feeling isolated and lonely. A sense of gratitude might not be something you are naturally feeling right now but if you find small things that you appreciate then you might notice these feelings become easier and more natural as you create new neural pathways in your brain. Having a daily gratitude practice has also been shown to help with sleep quality.[17]

We know that stress weakens our immune system, and we know that focusing on stress increases our stress, so how about focusing on something good? Giving thanks to someone or something, no matter how big or small. We always end class by giving thanks because from my experience the more we give thanks the easier it is to be thankful and sometimes it can remind us that even though we don't think we have anything to be grateful for, actually we do. An easy way to start to practise gratitude is to begin to write down each day something you are grateful for. You can start a gratitude journal that you can always reflect back on when you have feelings of being disconnected or lonely and remind yourself of the things you feel grateful for. Start small as big acorns can grow into big oak trees. Start with one thing you feel thankful for and then build on that to maybe two or three things a day. See if the feelings grow.

The heart is like a garden: it can grow compassion or fear, resentment or love. What seeds will you plant there?[18]

What you might start to experience is that with gratitude comes a sense of joy or contentment. In *Radical Remission: Surviving Cancer Against All Odds*, Kelly A Turner describes positive emotions as 'rocket fuel for your immune system' because we know our body has a better ability to repair and heal when it has the opportunity to move into 'rest and digest' mode and move out of 'fight or flight'.[19]

Mantra for gratitude

One of the oldest mantras is the **gayatri mantra**, which gives thanks to the sun that is forever giving and never receiving. The sun is seen as the source and inspiration of the universe, yet we rarely give appreciation to the sun and what it means in our lives. Chanting or meditating on the gayatri mantra asks the infinite light to guide us, shine through us and enlighten us. We often have this chant in the final relaxation of our yoga classes. You can hear the gayatri mantra on my website (vickyfox-yoga.com).

Om Bhur Bhuvaḥ Swaḥ
Tat-savitur Vareñyaṃ
Bhargo Devasya Dheemahi
Dhiyo Yonaḥ Prachodayāt.

Joint pain

A joint is where two bones in the body meet. The bones do not actually touch each other but are held together by ligaments and then muscles that attach to the bones via tendons. Most moveable joints in the body are synovial, which means they are encased in a joint capsule that secretes synovial fluid. You can think of the synovial fluid as a lubricant like WD40 that you might use to make the hinges of a door move more easily.

When we move a joint through its full range of motion, as we can do in yoga, we lubricate it. We move the articulating surface of the bone, the cartilage, around in the synovial fluid. This helps to keep the joints healthy as it improves the flow of vital nutrition to them.

It is important to start with warming up the smaller joints like fingers and toes first before moving up the body towards the larger joints like hips and shoulders. In yoga for cancer, we do a combination of dynamic poses, which warms up the joints to prepare them for any static poses which we will hold for a few breaths.

Joint pain can be due to any hormone therapy or surgery which creates a decrease in oestrogen levels; it may also be due to types of chemo or cancer that are near or in a joint; blood cancers can also cause pain in the joints. Inflammation in the joints can also cause bone or joint pain.

When we think of flexibility, we are really looking at the range of motion we have around a particular joint. Some joints are designed for mobility, like our shoulders, and some, like our hips, are designed for stability. The shoulder is a shallow joint that allows us to move our arms around in directions that permit us to wash our hair, reach up into cupboards or zip or button something behind our back. The hip joint is a much deeper ball-and-socket joint than the shoulder. This allows it to support the weight of the body and hold the thigh bone in place when we walk. The knee is a hinge joint which allows us to bend and straighten it, but it doesn't have the same range of motion as the shoulder or hip.

With joint mobility we also need to consider that injuries, or conditions like osteoarthritis, may also limit our range of motion, and this may be completely unrelated to cancer. Osteoarthritis is where the cartilage in the joints gradually wears down leading to inflammation in the joints. The inflammation can reduce the range of motion due to the fluid in the joint building up and limiting movement. It may also be pain that restricts us from moving our joint through its range of motion. In some conditions, like a ligament tear, you will need to seek specialist care to help the area to heal but some conditions, including osteoarthritis, may improve with yoga.

As muscles and fascia (the connective tissue that runs through and around the muscles) can restrict the movement of the joints, it is important to explore how keeping flexibility in muscles and fascia can also help increase range of motion and decrease pain or discomfort. Muscles attach to the bones via tendons. When we stretch, we draw the two points of attachment away from each other and we experience a stretching sensation in the fascia. Once we finish stretching, the muscle returns to its original size. We will look at this again in the 'Osteoporosis' chapter (page 171) because this pull of the muscle on the bone stimulates bone-building cells called osteoblasts. So, stretching helps strengthen muscles and bones.

'Fascia' is the name for the webbing of connective tissue that surrounds every bone, muscle and organ. It connects and holds the inner organs in place whilst allowing movement. So, for example, when we twist in yoga the organs shift but then come back into place when we come out of the twist. Our fascia is constantly adapting and is rich in nerve endings, making it a conscious and adaptive tissue. When we stretch, it is the fascia that feeds back information to the brain. Messages from inside the body come from the fascia and pain is felt in the fascia. It forms planes that run throughout the body literally connecting the body from head to foot. You can have a collapsed arch in your foot and yet feel it in your neck so when you are moving your joints, you also want to **look at the body as a whole**. If we can release tension in one area it will have a knock-on effect somewhere else and if we release tightness in the fascia this can reduce the pull in tension around the joints.

Whilst you read this, just stop for a moment, and notice your posture. Years of postural habits can make certain planes of fascia very tight. Sitting with a rounded spine and head forward, as we often do when on our computers, can make the front of the body short and tight and the back of the body long and weak.

Hands, arms and shoulders

Warm-ups for small joints of the hands

These exercises are taken from Doug Keller's *Yoga as Therapy Fundamentals* workbook (2014), with additional credit to Zephyr Wildman for the 'fascia flossing' exercises. They are designed to open up the nerve pathways in the hands and arms.

- Form a circle with your thumb and little finger (see Figure 47).
- Hold on to your index finger and draw this finger back towards you as you press the palm of your hand away from you. Try to maintain the circle between the thumb and the little finger. This stretches along the tendon of the index finger and the path of the radial nerve. You might even find you can start to straighten your arms (see Figure 48).
- Release your index finger but, keeping the circle between thumb and little finger, now hold on to your middle finger and stretch that finger towards you as you press the palm away from you. This stretches along the path of the medial nerve (see Figure 49).
- Final stretch for the path of the ulna nerve: hold onto your little and ring fingers and stretch them back towards you as you press the heel of your hand away from you (see Figure 50).

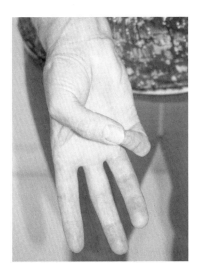

Figure 47: Forming a circle with your thumb and little finger

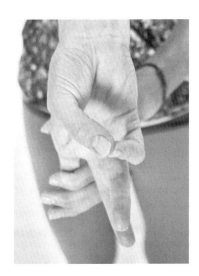

Figure 48: Drawing the index finger back

111

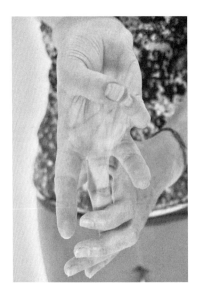
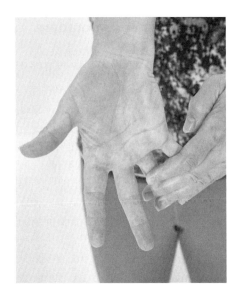

Figure 49: Stretching the middle finger   Figure 50: Holding on to the little and ring finger

Then release and shake out your hands and try any of the following small hand and wrist movements.

- Open and close your hands as if flicking water off your fingers.
- Hold up the flat palms of your hands to make stop signs. Then fold your thumbs into the palms and fold your fingers around the thumbs to make two fists. Circle each fist in one direction and then the other. Rotate your wrists like little propellors. Vary the height of your hands whilst doing this exercise.
- Move your hands up and down as if painting a wall.
- Conduct a small orchestra. Then start to make the movements bigger as if conducting a large orchestra.
- Wave your hands then turn your fingers down and into an upside-down wave.
- Interlace your fingers and draw a figure of eight with both wrists. Then change direction.
- Put your hands into a prayer position and press them together. Then press more with your left hand and then more with your right hand. Continue 4–5 times, alternating the pressure with the left and right hands.

Moving up the arms – elbows and shoulder joints

These next exercises also help to decrease the side effects of surgery and to get you back to your usual activities. Radiation may affect your arm and shoulder long after treatment has finished. So, movements to arms and shoulders will help keep mobility after radiation.

- Stretch your arms up in line with your shoulders and then bend your elbows to tap your fingers to your shoulders. Then re-straighten your arms.
- Tap your fingers to your shoulders and circle your elbows six times in one direction, then change and circle them in the opposite direction (see Figure 51).
- Stretch your arms out to the sides in line with your shoulders. Bend at your elbows and swing your forearms as if you are a scarecrow (see Figure 52).
- Then stretch your arms out to the side in line with your shoulders and turn one palm back and down, then forward and up. Then change to the other arm. Continue changing so you feel the movement rotate down your arms towards your shoulders, internally and externally rotating your arms. Feel each arm moving in its shoulder socket (see Figure 53).
- Interlace your fingers and, with your palms facing you, as you inhale raise your arms in front of you and as you exhale lower them back down. Repeat but notice if your body tries to help lift your arms up by the ribs poking out. Our body will take the path of least resistance, so if it is challenging to raise our arms, we often bend our spine and lift our ribs to get our arms up. Because we are trying to get rotation in our arms and shoulders, we want to soften our ribs down so that it is true shoulder mobility. Repeat 6–8 times. Don't push through pain, and notice if the repetition helps increase the range of motion.
- You can also turn your palms away from you and raise your arms forward and up; this might be more challenging (see Figure 54).
- Uncouple your arms. Often, we move our arms together so try inhaling and taking your right arm forward and up and your left arm down and back and start to circle the arms in opposite directions. This is way more challenging than it sounds and hopefully will bring a smile to your face as you try. It normally gets us giggling in class. Once you feel you have got the challenge, try changing directions!

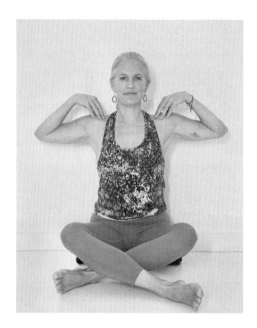

Figure 51: Tapping fingers to shoulders

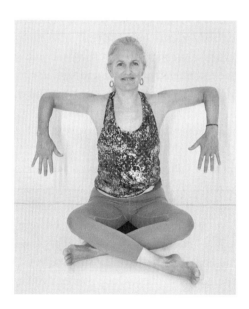

Figure 52: Swinging arms like a scarecrow

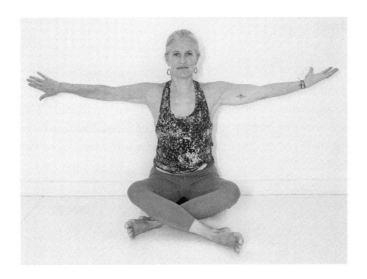

Figure 53: Rotating arms in shoulder sockets

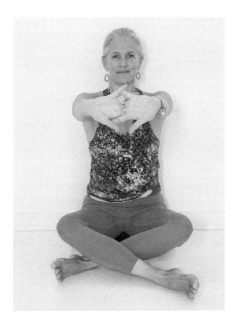

Figure 54: Raising arms forward and up

Legs and feet

Warm-ups for small joints of the feet

- Open your toes and then scrunch them up, making fists with your feet. Release and make the broadest, biggest feet you can. Repeat 3–4 more times.
- Interlace your fingers between the toes of one foot. This can be really challenging if you are not used to opening up your feet, so be kind to yourself (see Figure 55).

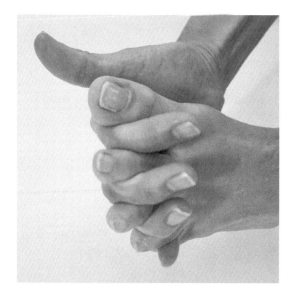

Figure 55: Interlacing fingers and toes

- Once you have laced your fingers between your toes, open your fingers wide so your toes abduct (move away from each other), then close your toes and try to squeeze your fingers with your toes, so your toes adduct (move towards each other). Repeat this a few times.
- Keeping your fingers laced between your toes, now move your toes forward and back a few times so you can get some movement in them and the small bones of your feet. (Lots of shoes are designed with the toes turned slightly

up so our toes spend a lot of time in extension; consequently it is great to move them into flexion and extension.)

- Then, keeping your fingers laced between your toes, can you circle your toes in one direction 4-6 times and then change direction.
- Release your fingers from your toes and stretch out your legs. Notice what it feels like in the foot you have been working on. Does it have more space compared with the foot you haven't yet opened? All we really have done here is released the fascia of the foot but it's amazing how different our feet feel after this.
- Repeat on the other side.

Releasing feet, shins and calves helps release the tension that might be held in our fascia. As we open up the small joints of our feet, this releases connective tissue that runs up through our body and through the diaphragm (our main breathing muscle). So, it is easy to see the benefit of small movements and the effect they can have on the rest of the body.

- Come down onto all fours and tuck your toes under.
- Sit back towards your heels. Your hands can stay on the floor or on your lap. Hug your heels in towards each other so you feel the big toe mound get a stretch (see Figure 56).
- Come back to all fours, place the top of your feet on the mat and just sit down on your heels (see Figure 57). Hands can stay on the floor or on your lap. There might be tension in your knees but there shouldn't be any pain. You can always place blankets or cushions at the back of your legs and sit on them instead of on your heels.
- To release the connective tissue at the front of your foot and shin, place your hand on the front of one knee and see if you can elevate the knee away from the floor. There shouldn't be any pain but it might feel quite intense as we don't often get a chance to stretch the front of our foot and shin. If you feel pain then back off out of the pose. See if you can keep breathing whilst you are doing the exercise and not holding your breath waiting for the pose to be over.
- Release and change sides (see Figure 58).

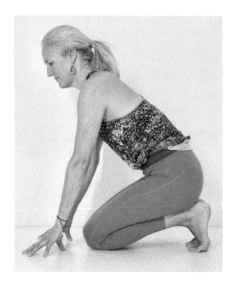

Figure 56 Stretching your feet

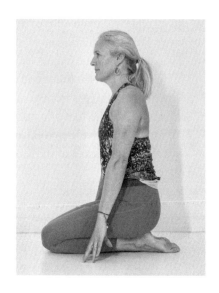

Figure 57: Sitting down on your heels

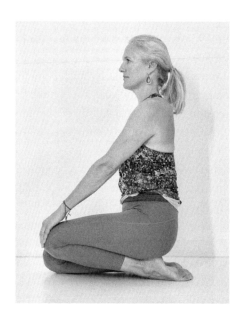

Figure 58: Elevating one knee from the floor

Calf massage

- Lie on your back and place the back of your right knee on top of your left knee and start to massage your calf by rocking the right leg forward and back (see Figure 35 on page 70).
- Work your way down your calf towards your heel. You will feel where the muscle starts to feel fibrous as it goes into the tendon.
- Then start to work your way back up on the outside of your calf, massaging all the way back towards your knee.
- If you find tight points, then you can stop and maybe change the massage by moving side to side or in circles.
- When you release, straighten out both legs and just notice the difference in them. One leg might feel more zingy or alive. One might feel more open. One side of your body might be easier to breathe into. Observe the effects of releasing the fascia on one leg. What does it feel like, and do you sense any openings in other areas of your body?
- Repeat on the left leg.

Stretch for the front of the feet and ankles

I love this standing fascia stretch for the front of the foot but if you are losing your toenails or experience pain in the toenail beds then I would skip this for the moment as it involves placing the toenails onto a blanket.

- If this is okay for your toenails, then from standing bend both knees and take your right foot back and place the front of the foot on a blanket.
- Without leaning forward start to straighten both legs.
- You should feel a stretch through the front of the right foot. If you don't experience a stretch, then bend both knees and slide your right foot a little further back and straighten both legs as though you are pressing up towards the ceiling (see Figures 59 and 60).
- You could also add on circling the right ankle in one direction and then the other while keeping the front of the right foot pressed against the blanket.
- Repeat on the left foot.

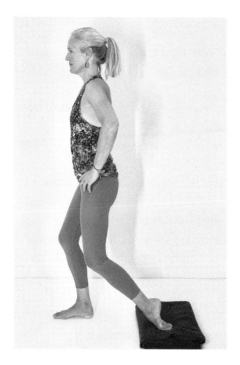

Figure 59: Bending knee in fascia stretch   Figure 60: Straightening leg
in fascia stretch

Calf raises

- Stand so that your feet feel comfortably placed under your hip sockets in **tadasana** (mountain pose). Soften your knees so you don't lock out your legs. Feel your feet. Notice if you are heavier in one foot that the other; if you are, press with your heavier foot to put weight into your lighter foot. Try to have a sense of evenness in both feet.
- Interlace your fingers and, as you **inhale**, elevate your heels and arms. **Exhale** and lower your heels and arms back down. Your heels might want to splay out so keep them hugging in towards each other. Repeat 4–5 times (see Figures 61 and 62).
- Try also calf raises with your toes turned out; on **inhale** elevate your heels and on **exhale** lower them.

- Or calf raises with toes turned in; on **inhale** elevate your heels and on **exhale** lower them.

Arms and legs together

Warrior II

- Step your feet wide. Turn your right toes out 90° and pick up your left heel and turn it slightly out. Press down through both feet and feel that there is even weight in both legs and feet. Keep that as you start to bend your right knee. When you look down at your knee is it over your ankle and not over your toes? If your knee goes too far forward over your toes it can put pressure on the kneecap (patella). You may find you need to lengthen the space between your right and left feet so that the knee doesn't go beyond the ankle.
- It may be that your knee doesn't go as far as being over your ankle and that this feels like hard work so it will be something you are working towards but perhaps not today.
- **Inhale**. Turn your palms forward and raise your arms out to the sides, going towards being in line with your shoulders (see Figure 63).
- **Exhale**. Lower your arms and straighten your leg (see Figure 64).
- **Inhale**. Bend your right knee and raise your arms, maybe taking them above shoulder height. Move in a pain-free range of motion.
- **Exhale**. Straighten your right leg and lower your arms back down.
- **Inhale**. Bend your front knee and raise your arms, maybe taking them further than before.
- **Exhale**. Straighten your leg and lower your arms back down.
- **Inhale**. Bend your front knee and raise your arms, maybe taking them further.
- **Exhale**. Straighten your leg and lower your arms back down.

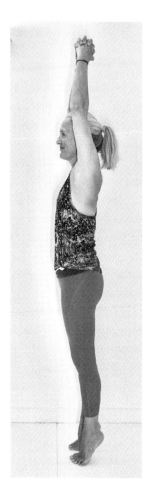

Figure 61: Elevating heels and arms

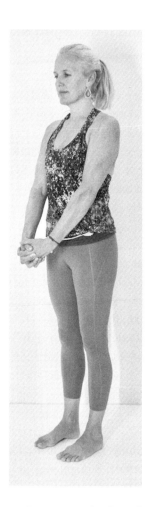

Figure 62: Lowering heels and arms

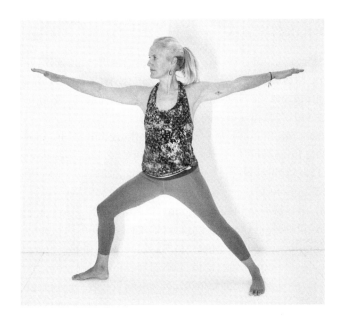

Figure 63: Warrior II – raising your arms, bending knee

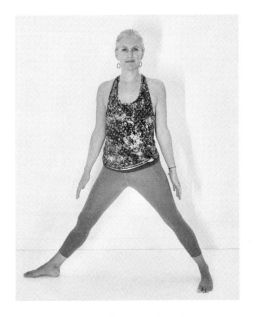

Figure 64: Warrior II – straightening your leg

Warrior II with hand movements

- This time as you **inhale** come into warrior II with your arms in line with your shoulders. Make a stop sign with your hands. Your fingers should be pointed to the ceiling and the heels of your hands pressed away from you. Take a breath in and a breath out (see Figure 65).
- Then close your thumb into your hand, followed by your index finger, middle finger, ring finger and little finger. Then turn the knuckles down towards the floor and press through the backs of your hands. Take a breath in and a breath out (see Figure 66).
- Then roll your arms and hands up towards the ceiling so you externally rotate your arms. Press out through the backs of your hands. Then release your little finger, ring finger, middle finger, index finger and thumb and press the palms out in an upside-down stop sign. Take a breath in and a breath out.
- Release and straighten your front (right) leg as you lower your arms back down.
- Repeat on the left side.

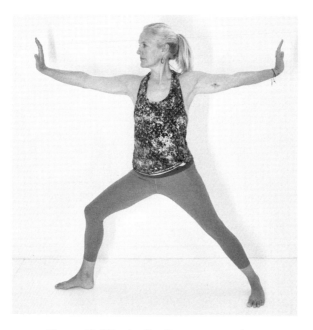

Figure 65: Warrior II – fingers pointed up

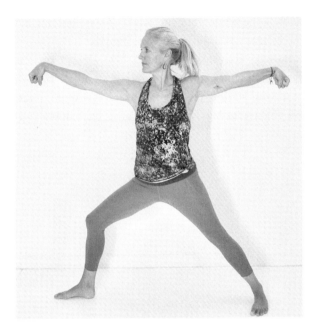

Figure 66: Warrior II – fingers pointed down

Tadasana

- Step your feet back together, put your hands on your hips and circle your hips five times in one direction, then five times in the opposite direction.
- Bend your knees and bring your hands to your knees and circle your knees five times in one direction and five times in the opposite direction.
- Standing in **tadasana**, bring your weight onto your right foot and, picking up your left knee, draw circles with it three times in one direction and then three times in the other direction. If balance evades you today, stand close to a wall or with a hand on a chair for support.
- Repeat with the right knee.

Horse stance

- Step your feet wide and turn your toes out. Feel the crown of your head over your pelvis and your spine long. Bend your knees coming into the **horse stance** (it looks like you are sitting on a wide cart horse) and then bend your elbows and tuck them into your sides as if you are holding a tray. Imagine that the tray is heavy, so you aren't working your biceps but maybe feel your large back muscles activated to hold the 'heavy tray' (see Figure 67).

- As you inhale, pull your hands away from each other, and as you exhale, come back to your starting position. Repeat a few more times (see Figure 68).
- **Inhale**, straighten your legs, lower your arms back down and release out of the pose.

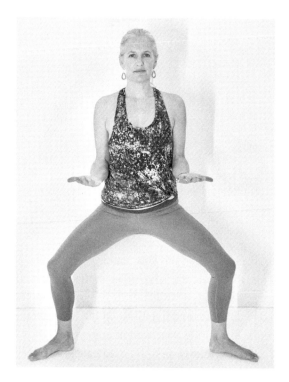

Figure 67: Horse stance – holding a tray

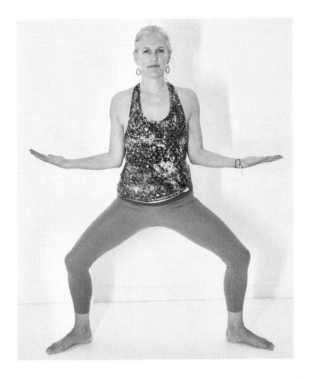

Figure 68: Horse stance – pulling hands away from each other

Twisted horse stance

- Bending your knees, come into the horse stance and, taking your hands onto your thighs, press down with your hands to lengthen your spine. Your spine should feel flat and long (neutral).
- **Inhale** and lengthen your spine.
- **Exhale** and drop your right shoulder forward and look to the left.
- **Inhale** and move back to the centre.
- **Exhale** and drop your left shoulder forward and gaze to the right. Feel the twist in your upper body and not into your lower back (see Figures 69 and 70).
- Repeat a few more times to each side.

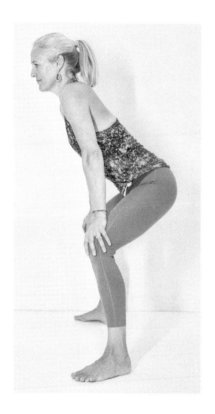
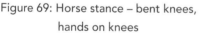
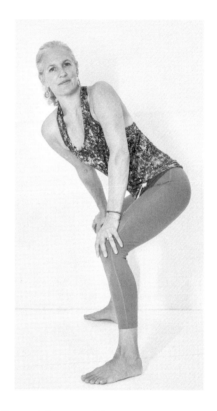

Figure 69: Horse stance – bent knees, hands on knees

Figure 70: Twisted horse stance – turning to the left

Arm swing

- **Inhale**, press down through your feet and use your leg strength to come back up to stand.
- **Exhale**, step your feet hip-distance apart and allow your arms to swing to the left and right. As your **arms swing** to the right, lift your left heel and as they swing to the left, lift your right heel.
- You can change the height of your arms to feel movement higher or lower in your spine.
- You can allow your hands to swing behind you and gently tap your lower back on the left and then the right. Stimulate the back of your body with your tapping.

Malasana

- Roll up a blanket or towel and, with your heels elevated on it, **inhale** and then, as you **exhale**, bend your knees and lower down towards a 'pain-free squat'.
- **Inhale** as you come back up using your legs and not your lower back; **exhale** as you lower back down.
- Repeat a few times and then come down towards a squat, **malasana**. Take a few breaths here (see Figure 71).
- If this doesn't work for your knees, then put something under your bottom or sit down on the floor, feet wide and knees bent and hug your right knee with your right hand and your left knee with your left hand or, for more support, take your hands behind you and press down into the floor to lengthen your spine, feeling the back of your ribs lift up and away from your lower back (see Figure 72).
- Then lower your bottom to the floor. Separate your feet and turn out your toes.

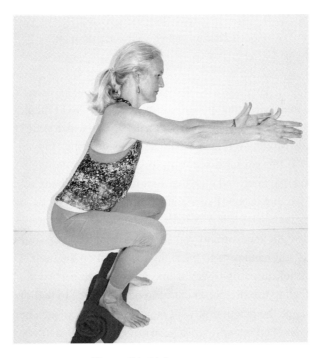

Figure 71: Malasana squat

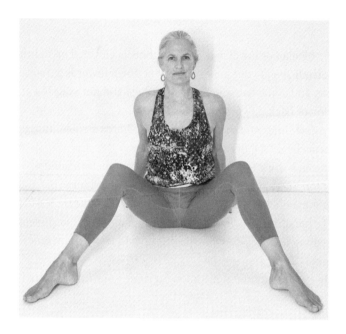

Figure 72: Alternative to malasana squat

Windscreen wiper

- From the malasana squat position bring your bottom to the floor and, keeping your knees bent and toes turned out, windscreen-wiper your knees from side to side Moving our knees from side to side brings movement into our hip joints. If this causes discomfort to your hips, try doing just one leg at a time. Bend one knee and tuck that foot towards your body as you move the opposite leg that is bent like a windscreen wiper.
- Then pause when your leg(s) go(es) to the right (see Figure 73).
- Take your right hand behind you so it is bearing most of your weight as you reach your left hand over to the right and rest it on the floor.
- Walk your left fingertips away from you (see Figure 74) and observe where you are feeling the stretch. There is no perfect place to feel the stretch so you might change the position of your hands to see if you get a better stretch in the hip areas. You may prefer to keep your hands close to your body or to walk them away and try walking them out at different angles.

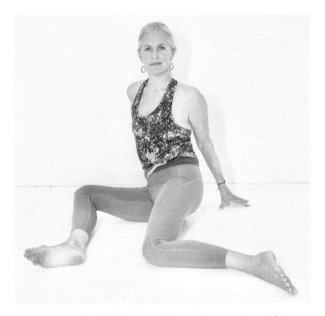

Figure 73: Windscreen wiper – legs to the right

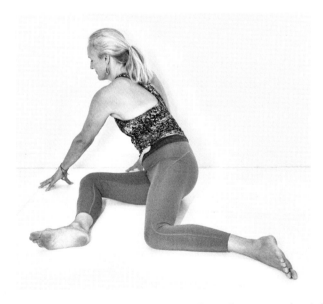

Figure 74: Windscreen wiper – legs to the right, turn to the right

- Take 5 breaths here and then bring your knees up and walk your hands back so that they are supporting you as you windscreen-wiper your knees to the opposite side.
- With your legs to the left (see Figure 75), keep your left hand behind you so it is bearing most of your weight as you reach your right hand over to the left and rest it on the floor. Walk your right fingertips away from you behind you and to the left. Move your hands away from your body and then maybe back in towards it, changing the angle of your arms to explore whether you get a better stretch with different positions of your arms, and observe where you are feeling the stretch (see Figure 76).
- Straighten your legs out in front of you. Wiggle your toes and circle your ankles in one direction for a few rounds and then in the opposite direction for a few more rounds. Then tap the mat or floor with the backs of your legs.

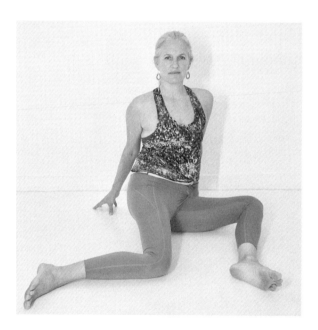

Figure 75: Windscreen wiper – legs to the left

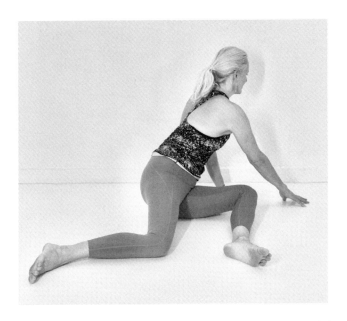

Figure 76: Windscreen wiper – legs to the left, turn to the left

To finish

Savasana

Finish by taking up a restorative pose or coming into savasana. Turn your toes in and out a few times and then allow your legs to 'plop' and relax on the mat.

Mudra for joints

You could add a mudra with your hands whilst in savasana. The **joint mudra** is the right-hand thumb to ring finger and left-hand thumb to middle finger; this is said to balance energy into the joints (see Figure 77).

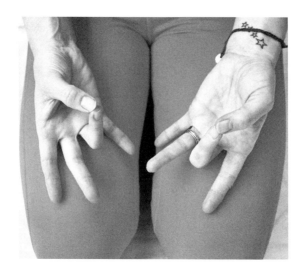

Figure 77: The joint mudra

Joint space relaxation

Guide your energy down to your toes and invite more space into your toes and feet. Sense your toes drifting away from your feet like little boats floating out at sea and feel the space in your feet. This brings awareness and invites more space into the ankles which in turn brings awareness and energy into the joints of the knees; moving up the body, invite space into the joints of the hips. Breathe down into your hip creases, feeling breath and energy moving down to your hips.

Sense the base of your spine and the spaces between your vertebrae; as you breathe in and out, your breath moves down your spine, massaging your vertebrae and the discs between them and lubricating each of the joints as your breath washes up and down your spine. Sense space in the joints of your chest and shoulders, space between your upper arms and forearms, space between your forearms and hands. Be aware of space in your hands, fingers and thumbs. As you soften and release, sense that you create more space in your hands, arms and shoulders.

Bring your awareness also to your jaw and soften your jaw. You could even yawn and open your mouth to release and sense the space at your lower jaw, gums and teeth. Allow your tongue to soften and broaden. Sense space in your upper jaw and allow the roof of your mouth to dome upwards towards the crown of your head.

Lymphoedema

We talked about the lymphatic system in the chapter on 'Immune system and infections' (page 101). The lymphatic system includes lymph nodes that work to filter and destroy nasties from our lymph and contain white blood cells called lymphocytes that fight infection. These nodes are what we often refer to as 'glands' that become swollen (active) when we are fighting an infection as they trap bacteria and viruses that they can't destroy immediately and, although there are nodes throughout the body, they are mainly in the neck, armpits, groin and abdomen . Lymph nodes are connected by lymphatic vessels and some of these vessels are very close to the surface of the skin. Sometimes lymph nodes have to be removed as part of cancer treatment and when this occurs there is a life-long risk of lymphoedema. The build-up of lymphatic fluid in the tissues of the limbs, neck and abdomen can be debilitating and painful and increase the risk of infection in affected areas.

The one-way lymphatic system relies on muscular contraction, flexion and compression, respiration, arterial pulse pressure and the natural pull of gravity to maintain tissue fluid balance and promote lymphatic drainage. Yoga postures, dynamic movement and breathing techniques can all help with these processes. According to Cancer Research UK,: 'Research has found that exercise and movement can help to lower the risk of developing lymphoedema. Most of this evidence comes from research into lymphoedema and breast cancer.'[1] A research study found that 'lymphatic flow is 2–3 times greater when we exercise than when the body is at rest',[2] and this helps us keep the fluid in our lymphatic system moving back towards our heart, which is the direction we want it moving in.

We want to move slowly, building back strength safely and taking baby steps to build up the strength needed for more challenging poses. The sequences in this chapter will give you the opportunity to build back strength in a safe way. They can help reduce swelling in the legs, build back muscle strength to help the muscles 'pump' fluid around the body and focus on deep breathing as a way of moving lymph fluid. We can squeeze areas of the body and then release them to create a tourniquet effect of compression into areas of lymph nodes. This is stimulating and helps movement.

Lymph is embedded in the fascia. Tightness in the fascia can prevent the movement of lymph, so releasing any stickiness in the fascia is important to allow more circulatory movement within the body. The poses in the chapter on 'Scar tissue' (page xx) will also be helpful to stimulate the lymphatic system.

BKS Iyengar, the founder of Iyengar yoga, emphasised in his teaching that postures that open up the 'armpits and leg pits' will help the lymph nodes do their work of filtering and removing toxins and harmful substances from the body.[3] So, poses in the chapter on 'Joint pain' that open up the groin and the armpits (page xxx) will also be a helpful addition too.

If you are living with lymphoedema, be mindful of doing too much weight-bearing activity before sufficient strength has been built. The advice is to start slow, with poses like four-point kneeling (page 109), before transitioning to more challenging weight-bearing poses. You can move dynamically, coming in and out of poses, so that you can take the weight off your arms. You should stop if your arms feel heavy, achy or tired.

As the lymphatic system is working less efficiently in people living with lymph-oedema, they are more susceptible to cellulitis. According to the Lymphoedema Support Network: 'Cellulitis is a sudden, non-contagious infection of the skin, characterised by redness, swelling and heat.'[4] The advice from LSN is that cellulitis should be treated immediately with appropriate antibiotics.

Warm-up exercises

Start with your breathing

Full diaphragmatic breathing helps to massage the thoracic duct and aids lymph flow. This is easier to feel when lying on your back.

- Take your hands onto your belly and notice its natural movement.
- As you inhale, your belly rises/expands and as you exhale it falls/deflates.
- Inhale and see your belly rise and then as you exhale notice how it draws in

and slightly up. Sensing the internal movement of your breath encourages the movement of lymph towards your heart.

Mobilising the small joints

Mobilising the small joints helps to move lymph from the periphery to the centre. Your ankles and wrists can act like a pump.

- Flex and point your feet.
- Squeeze your hands into fists and release them.
- Circle your hands and feet in one direction as you breathe in and then in the opposite direction as you breathe out.
- Bend your knees and bring your feet flat to the floor so your knees point up towards the ceiling. Interlace your fingers behind your head.
- **Inhale** and open your elbows and knees (so the soles of your feet come together).
- **Exhale** and squeeze your elbows and knees back to point towards the ceiling.
- Continue like this for 4–5 more breaths, creating a pump action in the groin, squeezing and opening the lymph nodes in the groin and those in the armpits (axilla) (see Figures 78 and 79).

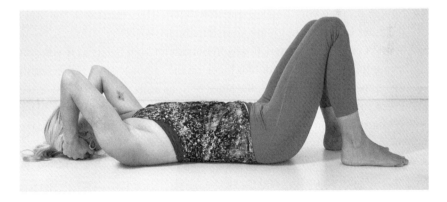

Figure 78: Squeeze elbows and knees together on exhale

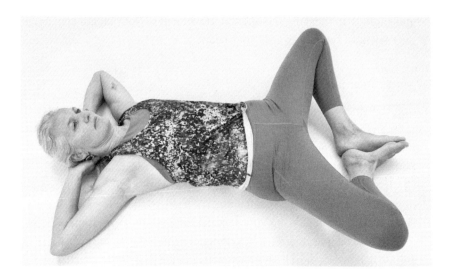

Figure 79: Open elbows and knees on inhale

Give yourself a hug

- Still lying on your back, **inhale** and move your arms out to the sides up to shoulder height.
- Stretch through your fingers, spreading them wide, then cross one arm over the other as if you are giving yourself a hug.
- With your arms still crossed, reach round with both hands as if you were trying to reach for the shoulder blade on the opposite side. If this feels too much then release and hold the sides of your arms instead.
- Press your elbows upwards and breathe in between your shoulder blades. We carry tension in our shoulders so imagine you are trying to massage your body with your breath (see Figure 80).
- Open your arms out wide and then change the cross of your arms so the opposite arm is on top, and repeat.
- Breathe 5–6 breaths in between your shoulder blades.

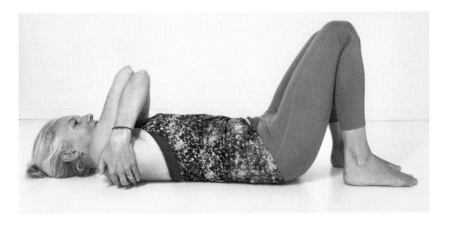

Figure 80: Hugging your arms

Exercise routine

Knee scissors

- Lying on your back, bend your knees and draw them in towards you with your arms by your sides. Lift your legs and arms up to the ceiling.
- **Inhale** and circle your raised feet and hands in one direction.
- **Exhale** and change direction; circle your raised hands and feet the other way.
- Repeat these movements 3–4 times, stimulating the joints of your ankles and feet and the muscles in your arms and legs, and allowing gravity to draw fluid back down your legs and arms towards your heart.
- Release your arms back down to the mat or floor and, as you **inhale**, separate your raised legs, making a wide V-position (see Figure 81).
- As you **exhale**, cross your left leg over your right and bend your knees (see Figure 82).
- **Inhale**, uncross and take your feet and legs wide again.
- **Exhale** and now cross your right leg over your left and bend your knees.
- Repeat 3–4 more times on each side.

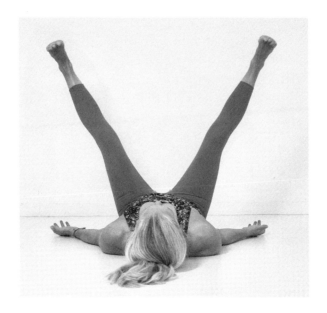

Figure 81: Legs in wide V-position

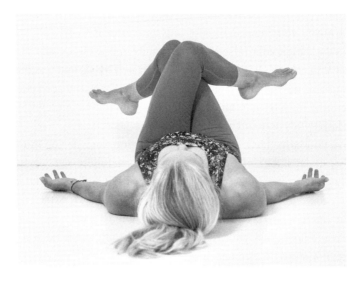

Figure 82 Left leg crossed over right

- From lying on your back, roll to the side that is more comfortable for you to roll onto. You might want to keep a stronger arm on top so that you can use it to press into the floor and roll up to sit. Your head will be the last thing to come up.
- Come up to sit on a folded blanket or cushion so when you cross your legs your knees are lower than the top of your pelvis.
- If you aren't comfortable sitting cross legged, then you might sit in a chair or extend your legs out in front of you.
- Check that your lower back isn't rounding behind you, but instead it feels like it is travelling forward keeping the natural curves of your spine.
- You should feel as if you can maintain this length of your spine even if you lift your hands away from the floor. If not, elevate your pelvis by sitting on more blankets. You can also support your legs with blankets/cushions or yoga blocks.

Opening up lymph vessels in your neck

- Turn your chin towards your right shoulder, then back to the centre; then turn it towards your left shoulder and back to the centre; repeat these movements a few times.
- Then bring your right ear to your right shoulder, then your chin towards your chest; then your left ear to your left shoulder.
- Then, lifting your chin, bring your right ear to your right shoulder so you are gently circling your head without dropping it forward or back.
- Circle three times to the right and then change the direction and circle three times to the left. This opens up the lymphatic vessels that lie close to the surface in the neck.
- Finish by stretching out through your body.

Sitting twist

- **Inhale** and reach your arms forward and up. Make fists with both hands (see Figure 83).
- **Exhale** and bend your elbows like rugby goalposts, and turn to the right, opening your hands (see Figure 84).
- **Inhale** and turn back to the centre and reach your arms up and make fists again.

- **Exhale** and bend your elbows like goalposts again but this time turn to the left, releasing the fists (see Figure 85).
- Repeat 2–3 more times on both sides.
- Come back to the centre and change the cross of your legs.
- **Inhale**, reach your arms forward and up. Make fists with your hands (as in Figure 83 previously).
- **Exhale** bending your elbows and pressing your forearms back to open up your chest (see Figure 86). Notice if this makes your ribs poke out. Soften your ribs in and breathe into the back of your body.
- **Inhale**.

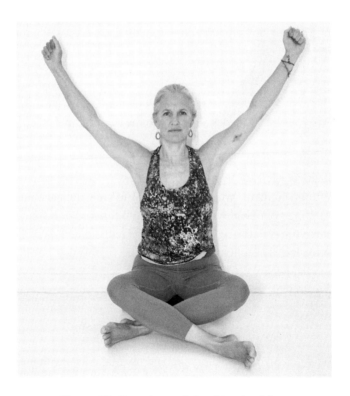

Figure 83: Cross-legged sit with raised fists

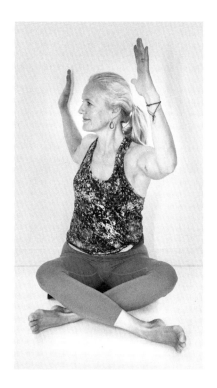
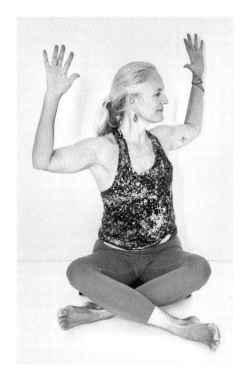

Figure 84: Cross-legged sit and turn to right with goal-post arms

Figure 85: Cross-legged sit and turn to left with goal-post arms

Armpit opener/side bend

- Remain seated cross-legged.
- Take your left hand to the back of your head where your neck meets your skull and lean to the right.
- Use your right hand to stroke from your left elbow to your armpit and across your chest towards your collarbone. This stimulates the lymphatic vessels that are close to the surface of the skin and gently guides the movement of lymph towards the heart (see Figure 87).
- Breathe into the left side of your body. Feel your breath expanding into the left side of your rib cage and all the way into your left arm pit.
- Drop your right ear towards your right shoulder and slowly lower your left

143

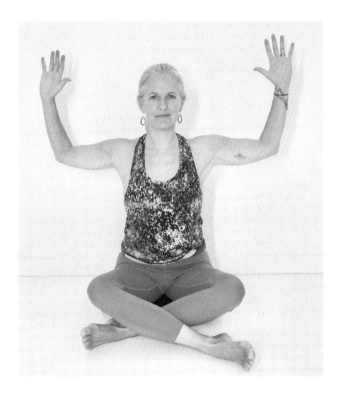

Figure 86: Cross-legged sit to centre with goal-post arms

arm to the left until you feel a stretch in the left side of your neck (see Figure 88).

- **Inhaling**, bring your right arm over your head as if you wanted to touch your left ear. Use the strength of your arm to bring your head all the way back up to neutral.
- Repeat on the other side.

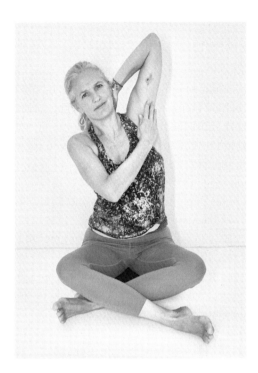

Figure 87: Cross-legged stroke of left armpit and collarbone

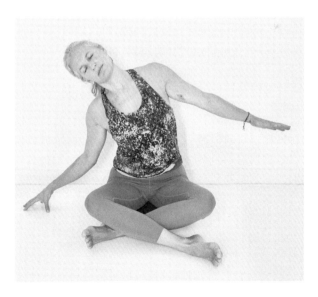

Figure 88: Cross-legged opening left side of neck

145

Groin opening and closing

- Come onto all fours. You can fold a blanket under your knees for more support.
- Your shoulders should be either over your wrists or slightly behind them. (I find slightly behind them an easier angle for the wrists that creates less pressure on them). Press the floor away from you. Feel that your spine feels long. You shouldn't be collapsing anywhere as you lift away from the floor.
- Extend your left leg back and as you do so, notice if you collapse on the right side.
- Hug your right outer thigh into your pelvis and lightly tone your belly so you support your lower back.
- Lift your left leg as you **inhale**. Lift from your inner thigh so your hips stay facing the floor (see Figure 89).
- Then, bending your left knee, take it out towards your left arm (see Figure 90).
- **Exhale**, circle your knee as you bring it to the mat or floor and press yourself back towards the Child's pose (see Figure 91).
- Repeat four more times on the left side.
- Change sides and repeat five times on the right side.
- From all fours come up to stand.

This sequence opens up the groin on both sides, creating some space, and then squeezes it to come back into the Child's pose. This change in pressure helps to stimulate the movement of lymphatic fluid, like a pump.

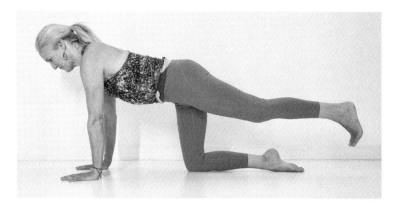

Figure 89: Lifting your left leg

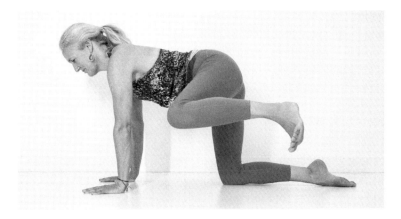

Figure 90: Moving your left leg outwards

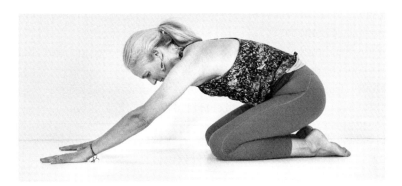

Figure 91: Child's pose

Tiptoe lifts

- If balancing is a challenge, you might want to stand near a wall or a chair for support doing this exercise.
- Stand with your feet a comfortable hip-distance apart.
- Interlace your fingers. This allows a stronger arm to support an arm with a limited range of motion if you have an arm that needs more support.
- **Inhale** and come onto the balls of your feet, raising your arms forward and up (see Figure 61, page 122).
- **Exhale** and lower your heels back down.

147

- Continue, but slowing the movement down so that it fits your breathing. You could even count your breaths in and out so that you move with these.
- Repeat 3–4 more times. Your heels might want to splay out so try to keep hugging them in. This helps to activate your calf muscles which help to pump fluid back up your legs towards your heart.

Dynamic warrior I

- Keeping your feet hip-distance apart, step your right foot back. Bend your left knee, checking that it doesn't go forward of your ankle and is tracking your middle toes. Keep your left knee bent and catch hold of the opposite elbow with the opposite hand (see Figure 92).
- **Inhale** and take your arms over your head as if taking off a jumper (see Figure 93).
- **Exhale** and straighten your legs, release your elbows and lower your arms down (see Figure 94).
- **Inhale**, bending your right knee, catch opposite elbows and take your arms over your head as if taking off a jumper again.
- **Exhale**, straightening your legs and lower your arms back down.
- Repeat 4–5 more times on both sides moving, with your breath.

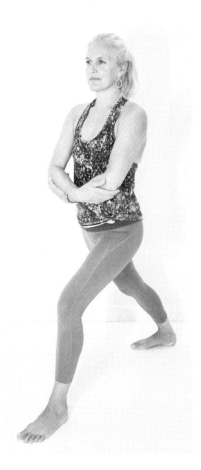

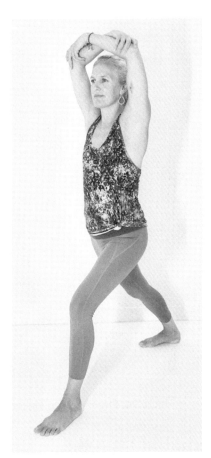

Figure 92: Stepping right foot back and catching opposite elbows with hands

Figure 93: Taking hands over the head (like removing a jumper)

149

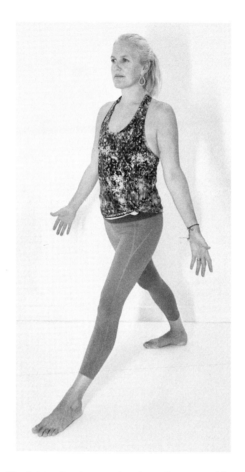

Figure 94: Straightening legs, releasing elbows and lowering arms

Eagle chair

- Place your feet a comfortable hip-distance apart so your feet are under your hip sockets. For more support you can always place yoga blocks on the outer sides of your feet.
- Bend your knees so you sit back into an imaginary chair. If that feels too low or challenging, sit back onto an imaginary bar stool instead, and extend your arms out in line with your shoulders (see Figure 95).
- **Inhale**.

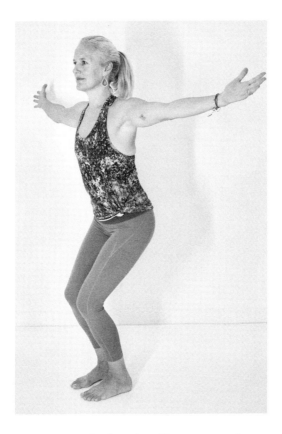

Figure 95: Eagle chair: bend knees, extend arms

- **Exhale** and cross your left leg over your right and your right arm over your left into a big giant bear hug (see Figure 96).
- **Inhale**, open your arms and uncross your legs.
- **Exhale**, cross your right leg over your left, and your left arm over your right, again into a big giant bear hug (see Figure 97).
- **Inhale**, open your arms, uncross your legs and come back to the centre.
- Repeat 2–3 more times on each side.
- For more challenge, you can stay in the eagle chair pose with the bear hug for 4–5 breaths before changing sides. For less challenge, keep your hands on your hips so you can just focus on your legs.

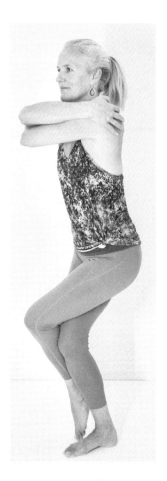

Figure 96: Bear hug with left leg crossed over right

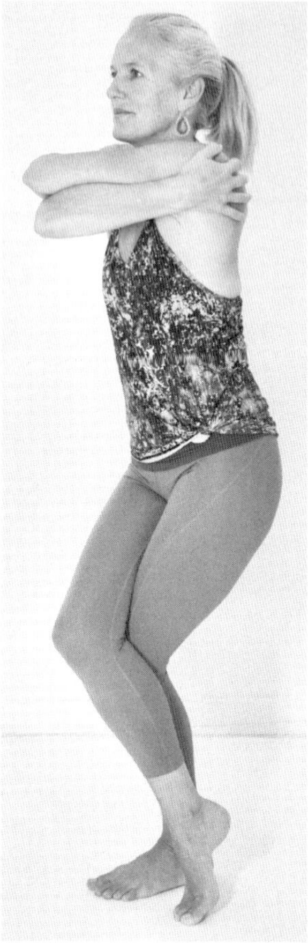

Figure 97: Bear hug with right leg crossed over left

Warrior II with archer twist

- Step your feet wide apart, turn your left toes out, lift your right heel and turn it slightly out.
- Starting with your arms down by your sides, press down evenly into both feet so you feel equal weight in the front and back foot.
- Elevate your arms in line with your shoulders or explore how it feels to take your arms slightly higher than shoulder level (see Figure 98).

- **Inhale** and look back at your right hand.
- **Exhale**, bring your right hand towards your left hand turning your upper body to the left (see Figure 99).
- **Inhale** and, starting at the wrist or forearm, stroke your left hand along your right arm and collarbone and bring your arm back to where you started (see Figure 100). This stroking stimulates the lymph vessels in your arm and encourages the movement of lymph back towards your heart.
- **Exhale** and sweep your right hand towards the left.
- **Inhale** and stroke your right hand along your left arm and collarbone and back to the start.
- Repeat three more times.
- Straighten your legs and turn your left toes in and right toes out. Lift up your left heel and turn it slightly out and repeat the archer twist on the left side 4–5 times.
- Turn your toes in and step your feet back together.

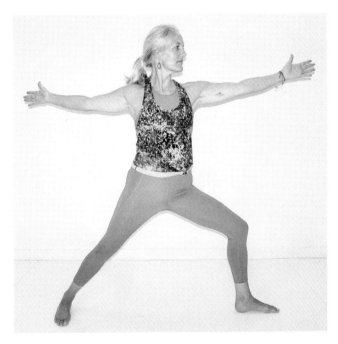

Figure 98: Warrior II with left arm forward

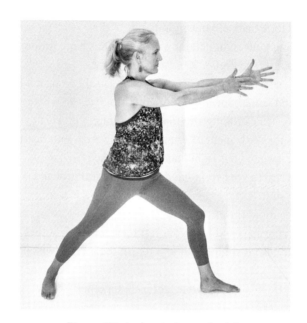

Figure 99: Archer twist to the left

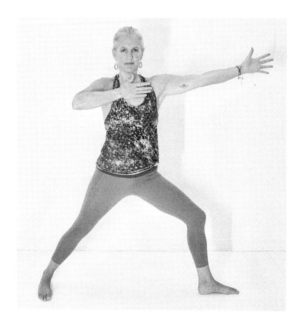

Figure 100: Stroking your arm and collarbone

To finish

Viparita karani

To finish we can come into the **viparita karani** pose with blankets. This pose is calming for the nervous system, and it turns the body upside down so gives it a break from its normal functioning of having to pump blood back up towards the heart. It can help to encourage movement of fluids towards the centre of the body to relieve swelling of the feet and ankles.

- Place two folded blankets near a wall.
- Sit with your outer hip on the blanket so you are close to the wall.
- Use your hands behind you on the floor to support you as you roll your sacrum onto the blankets and your legs up the wall.
- Push your hands into the floor to get your hips closer to the wall.
- Gently lower your head and shoulders backwards to the floor, keeping your hips close to the wall so that your legs don't lean but are supported and you feel your thighbones descending down into your pelvis.
- Stay like this for 5 minutes.

Legs-over-a-chair

An alternative to this is the legs-over-a-chair pose.

- You need to have two folded blankets, one for underneath your head and one that will go under your pelvis to keep it in neutral.
- Place a chair in front of you and sit on the folded blanket facing the chair.
- Take your legs over the chair so that your calves rest on the chair seat; lower yourself backwards onto the mat (see Figure 39, page 77).
- Adjust the blankets if needed so that your head is supported, there is space at your neck and your pelvis is in neutral.

Anytime exercises

Belly breathing

Breathe down into your belly. Can you sense your belly rise as you breathe in and fall as you breathe out? Can you sense the internal movement of your body when you breathe? Breathing fully and diaphragmatically massages your lymphatic duct, the largest lymph vessel in the body, and encourages the movement of the fluid back up to the heart. The lymphatic fluid passes through the lymph nodes to help filter out bacteria, waste and toxins. Lymph nodes also contain infection-fighting white blood cells. Once filtered, the lymph travels to one of two large lymphatic ducts just below the neck where they rejoin the bloodstream through a large vein (the subclavian vein named as it runs under the clavicle or collarbone) and carries waste towards the liver and kidneys which then gets released with the rest of the body's waste through bowel movements or urine.

Little and often

You can prevent the lymphatic system from becoming stagnant by using simple, easy movements throughout the day.

- Whilst you wait for the kettle to boil, raise your arms and make fists with your hands. Open and close your fists with your arms elevated to pump fluid back from your hands.
- Any time you are sitting, perhaps for mealtimes or to work, circle your ankles in one direction, then the other. Flex and point your feet to pump fluid back up your legs. Lift and lower your heels to stimulate the pumping action of your calf muscles.
- Whilst brushing your teeth, come up onto the balls of your feet and then lower them slowly back to the floor.
- You can also help to stimulate your feet by rolling a tennis ball under the them. Roll the ball from your toes to your heel and repeat again and again. This gently massages the lymphatic vessels. You can also roll the ball all around the sole of your foot, massaging your foot with the pressure of the ball.

For more support with lymphoedema you can go to the Lymphoedema Support Network (www.lymphoedema.org/). Golnaz Maleki is a wonderful yoga teacher specialising in lymphoedema and has videos on the LSN website to help with lymph flow (https://m.youtube.com/watch?v=25vT90oM6mk&t=2s&pp=2AECkAIB).

Menopause

Treatment for cancer can cause an early and sudden menopause which can be shocking and overwhelming. The symptoms of hot flushes, mood swings, vaginal dryness, foggy brain and fertility changes can be more severe than a natural menopause. You might also experience other side effects, such as feelings of depression, loss of confidence and fatigue, and the reduction in oestrogen can lead to a thinning of the bones.

The following practices can help support menopause symptoms by bringing movement and energy into the pelvic area and cooling and calming the body with breath. The practices in the chapters on 'Chemo brain' (page 53); 'Colostomy, ostomy, ileostomy and yoga with a stoma' (page 59); and 'Cramps' (page 69) will also be supportive as they bring awareness and movement into the pelvic floor. The practices in the chapter on 'Osteoporosis' (page 171) will help to strengthen your bones and those in the chapter on 'Joint pain' (page 109) will help move small joints that can become stiff or painful.

Cooling breathing techniques

Cooling breathing techniques, such as **sitali** or **sikali**, can help you take back some control which may help with the frequency of the hot flushes and make you feel less stressed by them.

Cooling breath

- Curl your tongue (like a straw). The ability to do this is genetically determined so if you can't curl your tongue, make a circle with your lips and breathe in as if you were doing so through a straw; alternatively, you can suck air in through the sides of your teeth.

- As you breathe, can you sense the cool air firstly in your mouth and then your throat?
- As you breathe out through your nose, can you visualise warmth from inside your body releasing out through your nose?
- As you continue to breathe in through your 'straw' (curled tongue/circled mouth) you can feel the cool air travelling down into your chest and as you exhale, any warmth from your chest being released out through your nose.
- Breathe cool air down into your abdomen and breathe out any heat through your nose. Sense the warm air as you breathe out.
- Breathe in through your 'straw'/curled tongue down into your pelvis and breathe out the heat from your pelvis, releasing it out through your nose.
- Continue for a few minutes until you sense your whole body being cooled by the cool air you breathe in and the release of warm air from your body through your nostrils.

Breathing down to the pelvic floor

- Come to lie on your back on your mat with a bolster or folded blankets by your side. Bend your knees.
- Raise your bottom onto the bolster or folded blankets. Elevate your pelvis so you take the weight of your organs away from your pelvic floor and start to breathe down into your pelvic floor.
- Visualise your pelvic floor broadening as you breathe in and doming and rising as you breathe out. The pelvic floor moves in conjunction with the respiratory diaphragm (that separates your chest cavity from your abdominal cavity and is attached around the rim of your rib cage) so, just by breathing, you are massaging and stimulating the pelvic area and encouraging blood flow into it (see Figure 26, page 60).
- Firming your belly, draw your right knee in and then your left knee in.
- Hold onto your right knee with your right hand and your left knee with your left hand and then let your knees separate away from each other (see Figure 32, page 66). Keep your pelvis neutral, so you don't feel like you are tipping to one side or that you have lost the natural curve of your spine (see Figure 31, page 64).

158

- Breathe down into your belly and sense your breathing moving into your pelvis.
- Observe if your breath or energy gets stuck anywhere. Can you breathe evenly down both sides of your body? If you feel that one side is not receiving the breath as much as the other, can you guide the awareness and breath into that side of your pelvis or belly?
- Stay for a minute, breathing down into your pelvic floor and, on an exhale, lower your feet to the floor.
- Press down into your feet and lift your pelvis so you can slide the bolster or blanket(s) out from underneath you. Allow your bottom to come down to the mat and just sense which areas of your body make contact with the floor.
- Feel the back of your head, the space at your neck, your ribs touching the mat, the space at your lower back and then finally the weight of your pelvis and your feet pressing down into the mat.
- As you breathe in, allow your pubic bone to move away from your face and as you exhale draw it back towards your face. The inhale puts your pelvis into an anterior tilt moving forward and as you exhale the pelvis moves into a more tucked or posterior position. Pelvic rocking helps to bring movement into the pelvis and lower back (see Figures 29 and 30, page 64).

Often when we spend a lot of time sitting, we can mould into the shape of our chairs, and this rounds our spine. In this rounded position it is more challenging to get breath, energy and movement down into our pelvic floor, which gets shortened when we round our spine. If we also sit with one leg crossed over the other, then this also shortens one side of the pelvic floor more than the other. Awareness is the first step to changing these habits so become aware of how you are sitting and any habits you may have of crossing one leg or rounding your spine.

Exercise routines

Supine twists

This pose creates space between your womb and heart, stretching and opening and allowing breath and therefore movement down into the belly and pelvis.

- Staying supine, find the natural curve of your spine where your lower back is not flattened into the mat or arching away from the mat.

- As you **exhale**, firm your belly to lift your feet away from the floor. For more challenge, your shins can be parallel to the floor.
- **Inhale** and bring your knees to the centre of your body and **exhale**, twisting your knees halfway to the right.
- **Inhale**, pause (no movement) and soften your chest and shoulders.
- **Exhale**, firming your belly, and, using your core, bring your knees up and over to the left.
- Repeat a few more times, moving on **exhale** from side to side; your core is supporting the movement (see Figure 21, page 48).
- You might like to stay for a 5-8 breaths with your legs over to the right and then 5-8 breaths with your legs to the left, breathing down into your pelvis. If you feel discomfort in your lower back, elevate your pelvic floor by putting cushions under your thighs, or between them so your knees stay hip-distance apart.
- Lengthen your top hip away from your face. Twists can be a big stretch into the chest area so you might want to change the angle of your arms so that you still receive a stretch or an opening in your chest but no pain.
- Roll to the side that is most comfortable to you. Press your top hand down into the floor and come up to sit, with your head coming up last.

Circling pelvis

- Come onto all fours with your shoulders over your wrists or just behind them and your knees in line with your hips. You might need a blanket or padding for your knees (see Figure 101).
- Then start to draw circles with your hips. Start small with your circles and then get bigger and bigger with your movement.
- If you need to take the pressure off your wrists, you might make bigger circles by guiding your bottom towards your heels so there is hardly any weight on your hands and then you can put the weight back into your hands as you circle away from your heels.
- Move in one direction for a minute and then change the direction and go the other way for a minute.
- You could also make these circles with your forearms resting on the floor or elevated onto blocks.

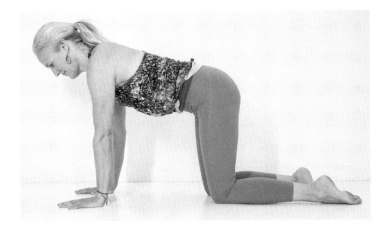

Figure 101: On all fours circling pelvis

Circling lunges

Leslie Howard taught me this exercise to get movement down into the pelvis and pelvic floor and I think it is fantastic.[1] If you take time to pause between sides and let your awareness travel to your sitting bones and hip creases, you might observe a difference between the two sides.

- From all fours, place your hands on blocks and step your left foot forward keeping your right knee on the ground. Does the height of your blocks allow you to keep your spine in neutral? If not, elevate the blocks so that you can keep your spine long (see Figure 102).
- Then walk your left foot to the left so that your hands are now on the inside of your foot. Turn the toes of your left foot slightly out to 45°.
- Start to circle your hips. Feel as if you are drawing circles with your left bottom or sitting bone.
- Continue with your hip circles in one direction for a minute and then change direction for another minute.
- Then step your left foot back to come back to all fours and pause to notice the difference between your right and left sides.
- You might even press back to the Child's pose to observe the sensations at the top of your thigh and the sitting bones on your left side and feel or sense if they are different from those on the right (see Figure 91, page 147).
- Repeat on the opposite side.

161

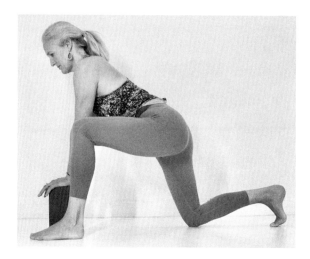

Figure 102: Hands on blocks for circle lunge

Calming poses

In *Relax and Renew: Restful Yoga For Stressful Times*, Judith Hanson Lasater describes hot flushes as the energy or prana moving from the centre of the body outwards, heating your skin.[2] She says that inversion draws the prana inwards towards the organs and away from the skin surfaces. This helps to cool the body back down. Restorative poses are also calming, and things feel more manageable when we are rested and restored. The side effects of hot flushes or mood changes can feel less overwhelming when we start to feel calmer.

Viparita karani with blankets

This pose, described and illustrated in the chapter on Hot flushes (see page 97) is calming for the nervous system, and it turns the body upside down, giving it a break from its normal functioning of having to pump blood from the legs back up towards the heart. It also increases blood flow to the pelvis.

Viparita karani with crossed legs

- Cross your legs at the ankles and rest your legs against the wall.

- Stay in this pose for 3–5 minutes.
- Change the cross of your legs halfway through the pose.
- Press the soles of your feet into the wall and push yourself away from it so that your legs now rest on the blanket and not the wall. Cross your legs at your ankles and rest your legs on the blankets for as long as you feel comfortable.
- To come out, uncross your legs and roll to the side that is most comfortable for you to lie on, then press down with your top hand and come to sit for a few minutes. Observe how it feels to be you right now.

Supta baddha konasana

- Using a belt or long scarf, create a large loop with it.
- Place a bolster or a pile of folded towels or blankets vertically a few inches behind you and sit in front of it with your knees bent.
- Have a folded blanket on the other end of the bolster for your head.
- Bend your knees out to the sides and bring the soles of your feet together.
- Place the looped belt or scarf around your sacrum/pelvis, like a belt. Then take it on the inside of your legs and pull the loop in front of you over your toes and underneath your feet so that the sides of your belt are on the inside edges of your legs.
- Now bring your feet closer to your pelvis and tighten the belt so that it is holding your legs close to your torso. Don't make the belt so tight that you feel a pull on your knees (see Figure 38, page 76).
- Lie back over the bolster and place your head on the blanket so that your chin doesn't tilt back, and you keep the natural curves in your neck. With your hands, slide your sacrum and buttocks towards your feet so that your lower back feels long. If you feel any compression in your lower back, you may need to slide a bit more away from the bolster to the end of the bolster that is towards your feet.
- Pull your shoulder blades away from your neck and roll the outer edges of your shoulders down so that your chest spreads from the centre to the sides. Let your arms release to your sides on the floor, spreading away from your chest, rotated outward, palms facing up.
- Place a cushion or yoga block underneath the outer edge of each leg.
- Close your eyes and rest for up to 10 minutes. Sense your breath moving

163

down into your belly and allow your shoulder blades to feel like they are sliding down the sides of the bolster and allowing gravity to open up your chest.

Yoni mudra

This mudra helps support the downward moving or grounding energy in the body by creating a downward pointing triangle shape with the hands. You can place this mudra on your lower belly so that your thumbs touch around your belly button area and your fingers point down and rest around the pubic bone area (index and middle fingers may touch). It is said in yoga tradition to regulate hormonal imbalances so can be beneficial when going through menopause (see Figure 103).

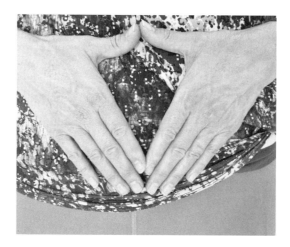

Figure 103: The yoni mudra

Nausea

Relaxation can help with the side effects of nausea. Focusing your awareness on your belly in the poses described below, take a breath in and breathe out through your mouth, making an audible sigh or sound. Our exhalation is linked to the calming side of our nervous system, the parasympathetic side. When we extend our exhale by saying 'aaaaahhhhhh', or by sighing, we activate this parasympathetic side and it allows us to start to feel more relaxed.

I should note here that we are not breathing out more breath, we are just lengthening the exhale. When we relax, our body has the opportunity to repair, nourish, heal and nurture itself; this is sometimes known as the 'rest and digest response' as the parasympathetic nervous system lowers our blood pressure, promotes digestion and eliminates waste from our bodies. It allows the body to go back to doing what it might have stopped doing through stress and cancer treatment.

Observe where you experience feelings of nausea. Is the sensation in your belly, chest, throat or mouth? Are you therefore holding tension in your belly, chest, throat or mouth? As you relax can you release your belly to allow breath to move down into it, guiding energy into the belly area, or maybe you can start to draw breath and energy into another area of your body where you feel you might be holding these sensations of nausea.

Notice if your mind starts to intervene and if you are being kind or judgemental towards yourself. Notice how we try to 'like' and attach to our sensations. Let go of your attachments (which does not mean you are indifferent to them or ignoring them) but acknowledge and understand them. Can you use your mind to catch your thoughts and then direct your breath to the parts of your body where you are holding any sensations that are challenging to you right now? Can you feel that your exhale is a way of letting go? Letting go of your breath but also letting go of tension in the muscles and organs of your body. Sometimes what we are also letting go of is our thoughts about our feelings and sensations, so try to let go of anything that doesn't serve a purpose right now.

Sense your body start to become heavy and soften down into your mat or bolster as you relax, almost as if you could make an imprint into the mat or bolster.

Calming poses

Supta baddha konasana

This pose opens up the front of the body, which increases the blood flow to the abdomen. This creates space for the organs of digestion and opens up the ribs to make it easier to breathe down into the belly (see Figure 38, page 76).

- Using a belt or long scarf, create a large loop.
- Place a bolster or a pile of folded towels or blankets vertically a few inches behind you and sit in front of it with your knees bent.
- Have a folded blanket at the other end of the bolster for your head.
- Bend your knees to the sides and bring the soles of your feet together.
- Place the looped belt or scarf around your sacrum/pelvis, like a belt. Then take it on the inside of your legs and pull the loop in front of you over your toes and underneath your feet so that the sides of the belt are on the inside edges of your legs. Now bring your feet closer to your pelvis and tighten the belt so that it is holding your legs close to your torso. Don't make the belt so tight that you feel a pull on your knees.
- Lie back over the bolster and place your head on the blanket so that your chin doesn't tilt back. With your hands, slide your sacrum and buttocks towards your feet so that your lower back feels long. If you feel any compression in your lower back, you may need to slide your body away from the bolster a little bit, towards your feet.
- Draw your shoulder blades away from your neck and roll the outer edges of your shoulders down so that your chest spreads from the centre to the sides. Let your arms release to your sides on the floor, spreading away from your chest, rotated outward, palms facing up.
- Place a cushion or yoga block underneath the outer edge of each leg.

- Close your eyes and rest for up to 10 minutes in this pose. Sense your breath moving down into your belly and allow your shoulder blades to feel as if they are sliding down the sides of the bolster and allowing gravity to open up your chest.

Viparita karani with blankets

This pose is calming for the nervous system, and it turns the body upside down thereby giving it a break from its normal functioning of having to pump blood back towards the heart. It also increases the blood flow to the pelvis and abdomen so can be beneficial for digestive distress as well (see Figure 42, page 86).

- Place one or two folded blankets near a wall. Sit with your outer hip on the blankets so you are close to the wall and then roll your sacrum onto the blankets so your legs move up the wall and your back comes to rest on the floor.
- Push your hands into the floor to move your hips closer to the wall. Gently lower your head and shoulders to the floor; keep your hips close to the wall so that your legs don't lean but are supported and you feel your thighbones descending down into your pelvis.
- Stay in this pose for 5 minutes.

Virasana (seated)

- Start seated in a kneeling position.
- Place one or two yoga blocks (stacked on top of each other if you are using more than one) in between your heels and sit back onto the blocks. Your heels will want to splay out so pull them in towards each other, towards the blocks. Can you sit on your sitting bones? If not, you can take your hands and gently draw the flesh of your bottom back to feel your sitting bones on the blocks.

The higher the blocks, the more space you will give your knees so it should feel comfortable. If height does not give you space and you are in pain at your knees, then come out of the pose (see Figure 104). Find a comfortable seated position where you are on your sitting bones and not rounding your lower back and sitting on your tailbone.

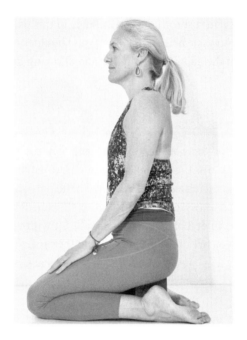

Figure 104: Virasana – sitting back on yoga blocks

Whilst in this pose (or any seated pose) you could also use the **pushan mudra** or **anuloma viloma** described next to help with nausea.

Pushan mudra

- Right hand: tips of thumb, index and middle finger are touching.
- Left hand: tips of the thumb, middle and ring finger are touching (see Figure 105).
- The other fingers are extended.

According to Gertrud Hirschi, this mudra 'influences the energy currents that are responsible for absorbing and utilising food' and 'has an excellent effect on general or acute nausea'.[1]

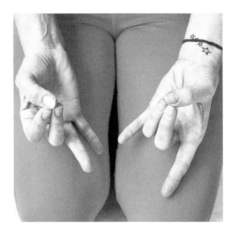

Figure 105: The pushan mudra

Anuloma viloma

This is also known as alternate nostril breathing and can also be balancing and calming.

- Take your dominant hand into a **vishnu mudra**, where the first and middle finger rest at the base of your thumb. Use your thumb to close off your right nostril.
- **Inhale** through your **left** nostril. At the top of the inhale close your left nostril.
- **Exhale** through your right nostril.
- **Inhale** through your **right** nostril. At the top of the inhale, close your right nostril.
- **Exhale** through your **left** nostril.
- This is one round. Continue breathing through alternate nostrils and notice if your breath starts to lengthen with each round.
- If you are congested, instead of closing your nostrils just visualise the air moving in through your left nostril and out through your right and then in through the right and out through the left.
- When you are ready to finish, exhale through your left nostril and then breathe in and out of both nostrils. Notice the effects of this practice.

The chapter on 'Digestion' (page 71) can also be supportive for the symptoms of nausea.

Osteoporosis

Treatments like chemotherapy and radiation attack fast-growing cancer cells. Unfortunately, fast-growing healthy cells, like bone cells and muscle cells, are also affected. Periods of time being inactive can also lead to the reduction in muscle tissue (known as muscle atrophy or wasting). Fatigue is a major side effect of treatment, and this fatigue can contribute to further muscle atrophy.

Osteoblasts are bone cells that build bone and therefore are responsible for bone density. Osteoclasts are cells that break down old and weaker bone. This balance gets disturbed as we get older, especially as women enter the menopause. Chemotherapy attacks the osteoblasts in the same way it attacks cancer cells and the osteoclasts become overactive which means more bone is broken down. This can lead to osteopenia (reduction in bone volume) and osteoporosis (decrease in bone mass). Without movement, decay occurs faster than growth, and extended bed rest can cause muscles to atrophy and bone to thin.

More than 80% of osteoporosis cases occur in post-menopausal women, who have lower levels of oestrogen, a vital hormone for bone density.[1] It is estimated by the NHS that osteoporosis affects over three million people in the UK.[2]

Bone grows and remodels in response to the forces that are placed upon it ('Wolff's law').[3]

Not only can yoga build strength in the bone by balancing and being weight bearing, but it also builds strength from the pull of the muscles on the bone. Muscles attach at two points on the relevant bones and when we stretch our muscles, they pull on the bones and stimulate them to create more bone tissue. Muscles also have opposing muscles that will be contracting in response to their opposite muscle being stretched, and again the tension stimulates the bone to create more tissue. We can therefore target our stretches to stretch the muscles in the areas where we want to strengthen our bones, such as the femur (thigh bone), the pelvis and the spine.

Many yoga poses involve weight bearing, which strengthens bones, increases spinal flexion and improves posture. A two-year study (Fishman and Saltonstall, 2009) found that the participants who had osteoporosis and did 10 specific yoga poses a day experienced improvements in bone density. Several improved enough to be reclassified to osteopenia.

It is also important that our bones are able to move through difference movement patterns, such as rotation, abduction, adduction, flexion and extension. Yoga-for-cancer poses move our bones around in all these various patterns. As mentioned above, when one muscle contracts and is flexing, the opposing muscle that is relaxing is extending and this pulls on the bones and stimulates bone growth, so any practices that move your bones around in different directions or stretch muscles will be having a positive impact on your bones.

Bone mineral density is only one measure of bone strength; it is the way that we measure bone, but it can be misleading. It doesn't take into account bone quality. What makes bones strong is the fascial network of soft tissue proteins (collagen) that calcium and other minerals are laid down on; these fibres crisscross each other in layers, allowing our bones to be strong and pliable, not rigid. The osteoclasts remove old and weaker bone allowing it to be replaced by better bone. If your bone quality is good, then you can have low bone mineral density and yet never have a fracture, but this also means that you can have high bone mineral density and still be at risk of fracture.

Safe practices to build bone strength

Aggressive or forceful yoga practice could put pressure or compression on the spine. Studies show that forward folds and twists can increase the risk of spinal fractures. **However this does not take into account the quality of the twists and folds.** We need to find a balance of strength and flexibility in the front and back of the spine and keep a neutral spine when folding or twisting.

Forward bend safely

- Try to move from the anterior tilt of the pelvis, folding from the tops of the thighs and not from the waist.

- The distance from your pubic bone to your sternum should not shorten when you forward fold.
- To help minimise any rounding in your spine I highly recommend using props. Yoga bricks, chairs and walls help to keep length in the front and back of your spine whilst you are moving (see Figure 106).
- To fold forward, first bend your knees as if you were sitting into an imaginary chair.
- Then take your hands to the tops of your thighs where they meet your pelvis and keep a long spine.
- Can you fold from here? How close to the ground do your hands go? Do you need to elevate the floor? Would a yoga block to bring the ground closer to you be of help? Would a chair or a wall help you to maintain length in your spine? (See Figure 107.)

You might notice in forward folds that this gives you a stretch in the hamstrings (the muscles at the backs of your legs). As these muscles stretch, they pull on the sitting bones and this stimulates the bones of the pelvis.

To come out of your forward fold, bend your knees and use the strength of your legs, and not your lower back, pressing down into the mat or floor to bring you up to stand. Keep your spine long and avoid rounding it up to come up to stand.

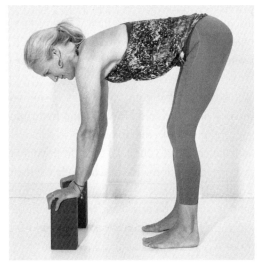

Figure 106: Using props when folding forward

173

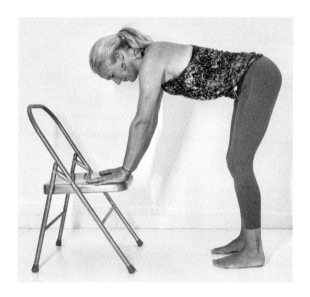

Figure 107: Using a chair to maintain length in the spine

Warrior III

Once you find a safe way of forward folding and keeping the length of your spine even on the front and back of your body, so your spine stays evenly long at the front and back which means you aren't rounding it, then you can start to add on some more bone-strengthening balances, such as warrior III.

- Form your forward fold with your neutral and long spine (perhaps holding onto a chair).
- Slightly tone your belly so that your lower back is supported, because as you fold forward gravity pulls the spine forward and by firming your belly you help keep the neutral curve of your spine.
- Lengthen through the crown of your head away from your tailbone. Then, feeling your feet, press down into your big toe mound, little toe mound and outer heel.
- Start to slide your right leg back without changing anything about the shape of your spine and feel how you now have more weight on your left leg. You might keep your right foot on the mat/floor or start to lift your right foot away from the mat/floor whilst keeping your spine neutral.
- Move dynamically, inhaling to lift your toes away from the floor and exhale to lower them down and repeat 3–4 more times (see Figure 108).

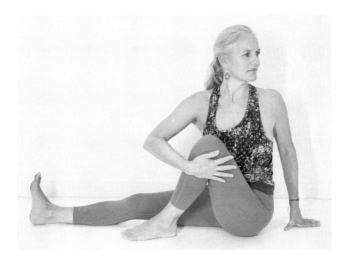

Figure 110: Twisting safely – arm gently hugs the leg

apply these principles to your everyday life so you move in a way that supports and strengthens you. Think about it next time you tie your shoelaces or pick something up from the floor.

Safe transitioning from floor to standing

- Coming to stand from the floor, first come up on to your knees (see Figure 111).
- Step your right foot forward, tuck the toes on your left foot under and place your hands on your right thigh (see Figure 112).
- Push off from your left foot to come to a standing position (see Figure 113).
- A more challenging sit to stand is as follows: from all fours tuck your toes under and walk your hands towards your knees. Then lift your knees away from the floor using the strength of your legs to come up to standing. You could always make sure you are by a wall for support (see Figure 114).
- Coming to stand via chair pose. From high kneeling, step your left foot forward, then push off your back (right) foot so you step forward with both knees bent and come into an imaginary chair. Use the strength of your legs to bring you up to standing (see Figure 115).

177

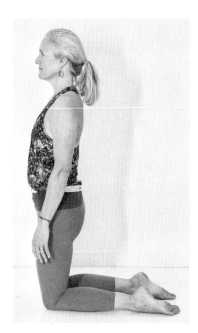

Figure 111: Kneeling up
from the mat

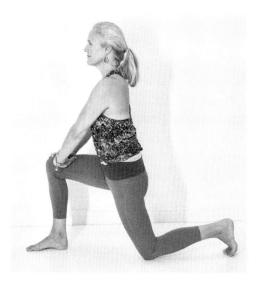

Figure 112: Moving the right foot forward

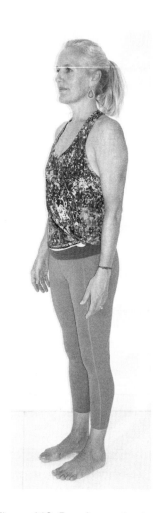

Figure 113: Pressing up to stand

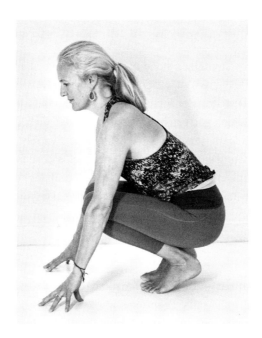

Figure 114: Walking hands to knees

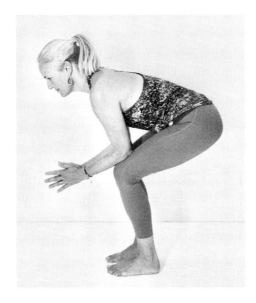

Figure 115: Coming to stand via chair pose

Balancing postures

Balancing postures help strengthen bone because when we stand on one leg that leg is now getting double the stress or weight of the body compared with when you are standing on two legs. That stress or force on the bone stimulates the bone to strengthen and renew. If you don't think you can balance, then think again because balance is a skill you can cultivate and relearn. Practising is key. Practise a variety of postures. Try them in challenging or distracting environments. You can pick a pose for the day and practise it whilst you brush your teeth (that will be 1 minute on each leg) or every time you boil the kettle. Notice your thoughts whilst you are balancing. Do you tell yourself that you 'can't do it!'? Or can you just tell yourself 'let's see what I can do today'?

Releasing the feet

Our feet are our foundations and are crucial to our balance. There is a link between lack of proprioception in feet and falls. Proprioception is our body's ability to sense itself, its movements and its location. So, connecting to our feet will help with coordination and balance. Our feet are designed to move on uneven terrain, but we put our feet in shoes and so they move as one unit. If we can release our feet, we will have more mobility in the joints and bones of the feet and we will become more connected to them and the ground beneath us.

When our feet are more pliable, the forces produced by walking or running are distributed and less shock goes into our knees and hips. The more time we can spend barefoot the better. This gives us the opportunity to adapt to different surfaces, challenges our balance more and is better for proprioception. The risk of loss of proprioception can increase with age or changes to nerves, joints and muscles, so the chapters on 'Peripheral neuropathy' (page 193), 'Weakness in muscles – building strength' (page 247) and 'Joint pain' (page 109) will also help.

The following exercise is a good warm-up to improve balance.

- Slide the fingers of your left hand between the toes of your right foot (see Figure 55, page 116).
- Squeeze your toes against your fingers so the toes adduct, and hold for a few breaths.
- Then open up the fingers of your left hand so your toes abduct and spread; hold for a few breaths.

- Repeat squeezing and opening your toes a few times.
- Then close your fingers around your toes and rock your toes forward and back a few times.
- Then circle your toes in one direction and then the other a few times each. Repeat with the other foot.
- Come onto all fours or four-point kneeling. You may need a folded blanket under your knees to support them. Now the weight is on your hands, knees and shins to stimulate the bones there.
- You can then add some movement by lifting your legs and arms. This will strengthen your bones as you move against gravity and will also help balance as you put more weight and stress on the bones that are holding you up. This will stimulate the osteoblasts to build more bone.

Dynamic sunbird

- Starting on your hands and knees with your shoulders slightly behind your wrists, find a long spine so your back feels flat, and you maintain its natural curves. Press your shins, feet and hands into the mat or floor and feel a sense of lift away from it.
- Slide your left foot back keeping both sides of your belly still working; check you haven't collapsed into your right hip and hug your outer right thigh in towards the midline.(see Figure 116).

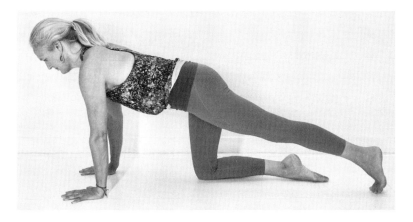

Figure 116: Dynamic sunbird – slide foot back

- **Exhale** bringing your left knee back to the starting position and repeat on the righthand side.
- **Inhale**, slide your right foot back and add on lifting your leg from your inner thigh so that your hips stay squared and don't open up to the right (see Figure 89, page 146).
- **Exhale**, lower your right leg and bring your knee back to the floor.
- **Inhale**, slide your left foot back and lift your left leg from your inner thigh.
- **Exhale**, lower your left leg and bring your knee back to the floor.
- **Inhale** and slide your right foot back with the option to lift your leg from your inner thigh.
- **Exhale** and lower your knee back to the floor.
- **Inhale** and slide your left foot back and your right arm forward, keeping a neutral spine; then lift your left leg from your inner thigh and maybe try lifting your right arm (or choose the option to keep it on the floor); see Figures 117 and 118.

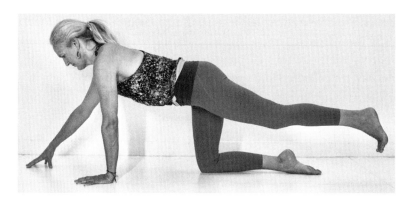

Figure 117: Dynamic sunbird – lift leg from inner thigh

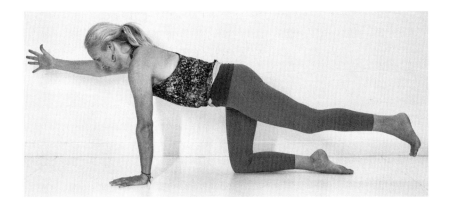

Figure 118: Dynamic sunbird – lift opposite arm

- **Exhale** and lower your right hand and left knee back down.
- **Inhale** and slide your right foot back and your left arm forward, keeping a neutral spine; and lift your right leg from your inner thigh, with the option of lifting your left arm.
- **Exhale** and lower your left hand and right knee back to the floor.
- **Inhale** and lift your left leg and right arm, then **exhale** and lower your left leg and right arm.
- **Inhale** and lift your right leg and left arm, then **exhale** and lower them both.
- Continue a few more times on each side.
- Tuck your toes under and walk your hands back towards your knees; optionally, you can place your hands on your thighs. Your heels will want to splay out, so you need to hug them in towards each other. Stay like this for a few breaths (see Figure 56, page 118).

Lunge twist

- Come up to high kneeling and step your right foot forward. Keeping your left hip over your left knee, draw your pubic bone towards your belly button to keep your lower belly toned and protect your lower back. Turn your palms forward.
- **Inhale** and raise your arms in line with your shoulders (airplane arms), keeping a long spine (see Figure 119).

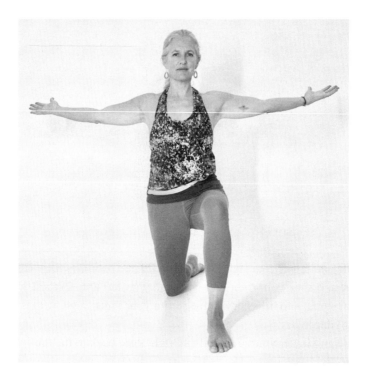

Figure 119: Lunge twist with airplane arms

- **Exhale** and, using your obliques (the muscles at side of your waist), turn to the right.
- **Inhale** and turn back to the centre
- **Exhale** and lower your arms.
- Repeat 3–4 more times, then step back to high kneeling.
- If it feels like too much strain on your arms, bend your elbows, bringing your fingertips to touch your temples and pressing your elbows away from each other as you turn to the right.
- **Repeat on the left** side with twists to the left (see Figure 120).

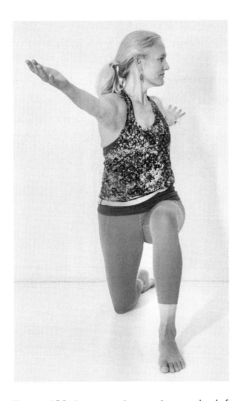

Figure 120: Lunge twist turning to the left

- To return to standing from high kneeling, step your right foot forward.
- Tuck your back toes under and place your hands on your right thigh.
- Press down with your hands and push off with your left foot to come up to standing.

Dynamic heel lifts with chair and block

- While standing, take a yoga block between your thighs and find the width of block that feels most comfortable. Gently hug the block so you feel your muscles hugging in towards the bone.
- Without dropping the block, draw your thighs away from it so you find a balance of your inner and outer thighs working.
- Check that you are pressing down evenly on the inside and outside of your

feet. Find balance in your feet and balance in your legs.

- **Inhale**, lift your heels and float your arms in front of you and up towards the ceiling (see Figure 121).
- **Exhale** and lower your heels and arms. Bend your knees as if you are sitting back into an imaginary chair (see Figure 122).
- **Inhale** and float your arms forward and up; then **exhale** and sit down a bit deeper.
- **Inhale** and straighten your legs to come up to standing. A more challenging option is to lift your heels as you come up to stand.
- Repeat 3–4 more times.

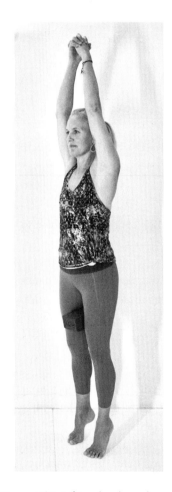

Figure 121: Lifting heels and arms

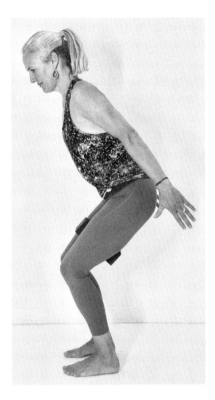

Figure 122: Lowering heels and arms and bending knees

Block balancing

This exercise helps us activate muscles when we are standing and balancing. We want to avoid collapsing down into joints but instead find space in our joints. Have you noticed that often we don't stand evenly or symmetrically on both feet? We often sink into one hip, collapsing into one leg, especially if we are standing for a while such as when waiting for a bus. We need to learn to balance with support and not collapse into our 'bus stop' pose, using the stabilising muscles of our glutes (buttock muscles). Again, props are really useful to help us to activate and feel these muscles.

- Using a book or a block to stand on, place yourself near a wall so that you have some support if you lose your balance.
- Stand onto the block with your left foot. Check that you can feel the big toe mound (the joint where the big toe joins the foot), the little toe mound (where

187

the little toe joins the foot) and the centre of your heel on the block. Your toes might come off the edge, but resist the temptation to grip the block with your toes.

- With your hands on the top of your pelvis, can you hover your right foot in line with your left foot until your hips feel balanced in relation to the ground? (See Figure 123).
- Then lower your right foot towards the floor and notice how your hips drop and you slightly collapse into your left outer thigh (see Figure 124).
- Press your left outer thigh in to lift your right foot back up to the level of the left.
- Then take your hands to your outer thighs (see Figure 125).

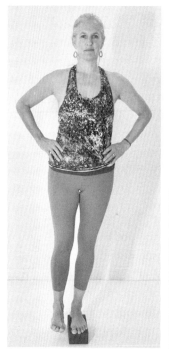 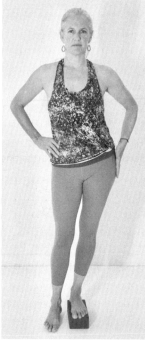 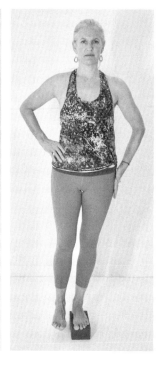

Figure 123: Foot hovering in line with the foot on the block

Figure 124: Hips drop and slightly collapse into outer thigh

Figure 125: Pressing outer thigh in to level hips

You might feel the area of bone at the top of your thigh in line with your pubic bone (called the greater trochanter of the femur). Now notice that if you repeat the exercise by pressing your hand into your outer thigh it brings your hips back to level. Repeat this a few times and observe which muscles you feel working on your balancing (weight-bearing) leg.

This exercise helps us just to activate our muscles so that when we stand, we are not collapsing into our joints but using our muscles to create space in the joints. You can think of these joints as being like a trampoline that is supported by the springs around it. If some of the springs don't work, then the trampoline will not function fully and will not be as stable. The same happens with our joints and we want all our muscles (our springs) to be working evenly to support and stabilise our joints.

If you continue lowering your left leg and lifting it back to neutral, you will feel the stabilising muscles of your glutes on your right leg working and therefore strengthening.

Finally, come off the block. Shake out your legs and use your hands to tap or pat the area where you felt your muscles working. Then repeat on the other side.

Tree pose on a block or book

- You can stand by a wall for support here.
- Step back onto the block with your right foot. Feel your big toe mound, little toe mound and heel. Notice if you roll onto one side of your foot; you need to feel evenly balanced on the left and right sides of the foot.
- Then, with your hands on the top of your pelvis, lift your left foot up keeping your spine neutral, not rounding forward or tipping back. When the top of your pelvis feels level in relation to the ground, we know that we are not actively shortening one side of our spine.
- Keeping your hands on the tops of your pelvis, bend your left knee and take it out to the left without your pelvis turning to the left.
- Can you feel your glutes working here? Take a hand to your bottom to feel if there is a firming of the muscles. Can you activate them, so they are working to externally rotate your leg?
- Then bring the sole of your left foot to rest below your right knee, or above your right knee if you want a greater challenge (see Figure 126).

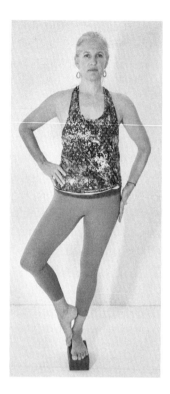

Figure 126: Tree pose on a block or book

- Notice if your hips shift to the right; if they do, hug your right outer hip in so that you are stabilising it and not collapsing or sinking into that hip.
- Take a few breaths in this position then release and change sides.

You could also try following the sequences in the chapters on 'Weakness in muscles – building strength' (page 247) and 'Scar tissue' (page 209) to help to build back muscle strength; we know this stimulates the bone-building activity of osteoblasts which then turn to osteocytes, cells that become embedded in the bone. The more we strengthen and lengthen our muscles, the stronger our bones will be. Sequences in the chapter on 'Joint pain' (page xx) will also help increase our range of motion and therefore our agility and flexibility and make us less likely to fall or more likely to be able to catch ourselves if we do.

Being mindful as opposed to mindless will also help with our proprioception and our balance. We often trip over things when we are not truly paying attention. Our mind was somewhere else, and we didn't notice what was on the floor or what our feet were doing. So, try balancing and staying with your breath. Breathing in fully and breathing out fully. It's easier to balance if you keep your gaze at the horizon so your eyes aren't darting about the room and gaze softly instead.

Notice your thoughts. Do you tell yourself you can't do it? Are you being kind in the way you are speaking to yourself? Would you say these same things to someone else? Can you put a hint of a smile on your face? Let the corners of your mouth turn up and notice how it feels when you balance with the addition of a smile. Sense the energy of a smile and the essence of joy behind the smile.

Restorative poses

Prithivi mudra

To strengthen your bones, with both hands lightly bring your ring finger and thumb to touch, letting your other fingers lengthen away from your hand (see Figure 127). In the Ayurvedic tradition, the thumb represents the element of fire which is great for transformation and the ring finger represents the element of earth, which is grounding. Bones, muscles, tendons and organs are seen as being earth elements, so yoga tradition sees that, by increasing the earth element, we help to create more balance in these areas.

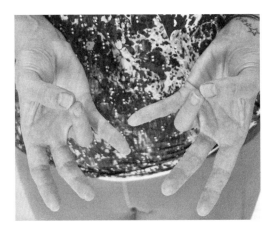

Figure 127: The prithivi mudra

As described previously, when we experience high levels of stress, we release cortisol and unfortunately cortisol breaks down bone (it blocks the osteoblasts) when it is chronically elevated, so passive poses that calm the nervous system are important too for our bone strength. Try finishing with restorative postures, such as those in the chapters on 'Digestive problems and discomfort' (page 73), 'Nausea' (page 165) and 'Menopause' (page 157).

Thank you to Melina Meza for your time to discuss flexion of the spine with me and to help me create safe practices.

Peripheral neuropathy

Peripheral neuropathy is the name for loss of sensation in the limbs, hands and feet; it can occur when sensory nerves are damaged during chemo and no longer transmit information between the central nervous system and the rest of the body. This is known as chemotherapy-induced peripheral neuropathy (CIPN) and can result in numbness, tingling, burning or pain, often in the hands, feet and legs. It may make it hard to balance if you lose connection to your feet; this can be very mentally frustrating as well as physically challenging because, if you can't feel your feet, the potential to trip or fall increases.

If we lose connection to our hands, we can start to feel disconnected and use them less; this can in turn mean that small movements become harder to do, like being able to button up shirts. This chapter focuses on practices that keep fingers, wrists, hands ankles, feet and toes flexible and strong to help prevent muscle wastage. The joint opening sequences in the chapter on 'Joint pain' (page 111) will also be helpful to get movement, strength and flexibility in the hands and feet. Nerves are held within the fascia (page 119) so the opening sequences in the chapter on 'Scar tissue' (page 209) and the chapter on 'Lymphoedema' (page 135) will also help, as they are focused on opening up the connective tissue that can get a bit stuck and limit the movement of the bundles of nerves within the fascia.

Get acquainted with your feet

I am really grateful to my anatomy teacher, Doug Keller, for focusing on the foundations of our feet and hands; it is through his trainings that I have learnt some of

193

the gems that I am able to share with you.[1] Our feet evolved to run around on uneven terrain, so they have lots of small bones that allow our feet to respond to the ground beneath us. Because we put our feet into shoes, they end up working as one unit moving around on a flat surface and their small joints don't get moved or manipulated enough. The exercises in this chapter are great for moving the toes and small bones of the feet, lubricating the joints, making our feet more malleable and therefore giving us a better connection to our feet.

I highly recommend spending as much time as you can in bare feet when you are walking around your home. This can help to make you more aware of your feet. When you are standing, notice if you tend to roll to one side of your foot. Do both your feet do the same thing or does one foot do something different to the other foot? If you are not aware of your feet, it can be good to get acquainted and feel the soles of your feet with your hands.

Find your big toe joint – where your big toe joins your foot – and feel the mound on your sole. Rub your thumbs around it so you can feel how big it is. Then feel the little toe mound, where the little toe joins the foot. Then feel your heel and rub your fingers around the sole of your foot where the heel is to feel how large this surface is. The two most weight-bearing points on your feet are the big toe mound and the outer heel and they support the inner arch of your foot.

When you are standing, can you feel the three points of big toe mound, little toe mound and outer heel? Try lifting up your toes to feel the big toe mound grounding. Then, keeping your big and middle toes lifted, lengthen your foot out and down through your little toe and sense how you start to ground down through your outer heel. Try to keep your big toe mound grounded and try not to roll to the little-toe side of your foot. Feel how connected your feet are to the earth.

Slide fingers between toes

Slide each of your fingers between each of your toes. This exercise gets the toes opening (abducting) and closing (adducting) and can be really challenging. The hardest part can be just sliding your fingers in between your toes. Try using the opposite hand to your foot. You might use your spare hand to help open up and create some space for your fingers (see Figure 55, page 116 in the 'Joint pain' chapter).

- Once you have your fingers in between your toes, squeeze your fingers with your toes and breathe five breaths.
- Then open up your fingers to open the toes and breathe five breaths.

- Repeat both squeezing and opening up.
- Then, close your fingers around your toes and rock your toes forward and back (flexion and extension) a few times or for up to 1 minute.
- Then circle your toes (circumduction) in one direction for a few breaths and then change direction.
- Release your fingers from your toes and just feel the difference between your two feet. The foot you have just opened might feel more spacious than the foot you haven't yet opened. You can do this exercise whilst watching TV or relaxing.

Fist feet

- Start from sitting on a chair. Look down at your feet and scrunch up your toes to make a fist with your foot. It feels like you are drawing your toes towards your heel.
- Hold for a breath and then release and repeat 3–4 times.
- Your feet might cramp. This is perfectly normal, especially if you are not used to moving your feet in this way. If you experience cramp, come out of the pose, wiggle your toes and feet and then come back into the pose.

Then do the above exercise standing up. If balance is challenging, or you feel very disconnected to your feet, try padding or tapping your feet on the floor to help to start to 'feel' them more. You can stand close to a wall or chair for support. Scrunch up your toes to make a fist, holding for a few breaths and then releasing.

For more challenge, from standing, scrunch your toes towards your heels and then see if you can shuffle your heels closer to your toes. You will feel your arches lift and the soles of each foot working. Pause for a breath and then release. You can repeat this a few more times and notice if you are actually moving forward with each repetition.

Strengthening fingers and hands

Finger press ups

- Sitting at a table or desk, place a tissue flat underneath your hand.
- Make a flat tent shape with your fingers so there is space underneath the palm of your hand (see Figure 128).

195

- Then scrunch the tissue with your fingers as you draw them in towards each other into a tee pee shape (see Figure 129).
- Then slide your fingers out away from each other.
- To make this more challenging you can repeat the same action on all fours. Then try to 'fluff up' your yoga mat with your fingers.
- One hand at a time, pull your fingers together, in and away from the floor or table so that you feel as if you are trying to pull up the floor/table towards you.
- Repeat 3–4 times with each hand.

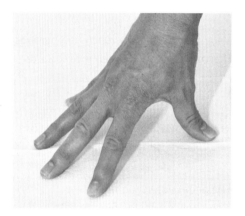 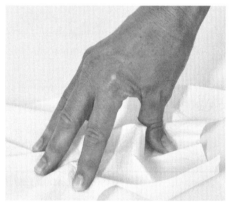

Figure 128: Making a flat tent shape with the fingers

Figure 129: Placing a hand over a tissue and scrunching up

Doug and Zephyr's fascia flossing exercises

The following exercise is designed to open up the nerve pathways in the hands and arms.[1] Refer to the chapter on 'Joint pain' (page 109) to follow the sequence of illustrations.

- Form a circle with the thumb and little finger of your left hand (see Figure 47, page 111).
- Hold on to your index finger with your right hand and draw it back towards you as you press your left palm away from you (see Figure 48, page 111). Try to maintain the circle between your thumb and little finger. This stretches along the tendon of the index finger and the path of the radial nerve. You

might even find you can start to straighten your arm.

- Release your index finger but, keeping the circle between thumb and little finger, now hold onto your middle finger and stretch it back towards you as you press your left palm away from you. This stretches along the path of the medial nerve (see Figure 49, page 112).
- Finally, stretch the path of the ulna nerve by holding onto your little and ring fingers and stretching those fingers back towards you as you press the heel of your hand away from you (see Figure 50, page 112). (Of course, you have to release the thumb-little finger circle to do this.) Stretch your thumb, index and middle fingers away from each other.

Releasing fascia from neck to hands

In the next exercise, first sit down and extend your arms out to the sides in line with your shoulders.

- Make a stop sign with each hand so palms face away, and your fingers point up (see Figure 130).
- Then turn your hand so your fingers point down and press through the heel of the hands (see Figure 131).
- Then repeat but reach one arm back a little bit behind you and turn to gaze at the opposite arm.
- Observe where you feel that stretch.
- Hold for a few breaths and then bring the arm back in line with your shoulder and repeat with the other arm.

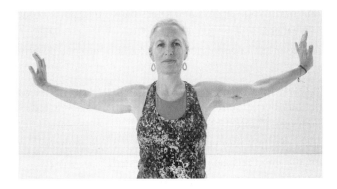

Figure 130: Palms out, fingers up like a stop sign

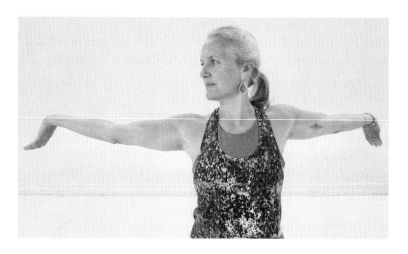

Figure 131: Palms out, fingers down, pressing through heel of hand

Groin and armpits

Releasing out the groin and armpits to help create some space in these important areas allows the tissue to release and the nerves that are held in the fascia to flow more freely.

- Lie on your back with your knees bent and feet flat on the floor.
- Interlace your fingers behind your head and point your elbows up to the ceiling.
- **Inhale** and open your elbows and knees out away from each other to the side.
- **Exhale** and bring your elbows and knees back up to point at the ceiling.
- Repeat 5–6 times.
- Then, drop your left knee to the left and keep right knee pointing up to the ceiling.
- Allow your elbows to drop down towards the floor and stretch your left knee to the left and your left elbow up and to the left. So, same side elbow and knee stretch (see Figure 132).
- Pause here, breathing into your armpit and down into the left side of your groin. Breathe into the space you have created.
- Take 5–8 breaths here then bring your left knee up to point at the ceiling and drop your right knee out to the right.

- Stretch your right elbow away from your right knee. Create a little side bend on the right side.

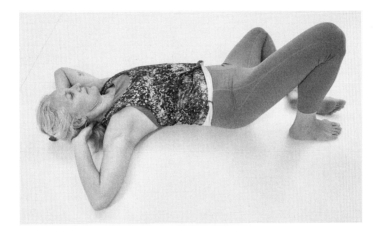

Figure 132: Stretching left elbow away from left knee

Referred pain

Referred pain is defined as 'an unpleasant sensory and emotional experience associated with, or resembling that associated with, actual or potential tissue damage'.[1]

Pain can be something that goes away after wounds from surgery heal but sometimes it is more persistent and can become chronic. With referred pain you might feel the pain somewhere away from the site of an injury. 'Nerve pain' can be a numbing or shooting sensation; 'bone pain' can be a dull or throbbing ache; some pain can be hard to pinpoint; and some pain is 'phantom pain' in that it is experienced in an area of the body that has been removed.

Pain can prevent you sleeping and can be all-consuming. Studies into yoga and pain reported that people who participated in a 75-minute yoga practice twice weekly for four weeks experienced great reductions in pain, muscle aches, time spent in bed and feelings of weakness.[2] A reduction in pain might make exercising more accessible and therefore give you the opportunity to reap the other benefits that a yoga practice can bring.[3]

A study in 2017 looked at the effects of pain on respiration (breathing).[4] It found that our breathing changes in response to pain: 'an inspiratory gasp with a subsequent breath-hold in response to sudden onset, acute pain, a sigh of relief when pain is removed, or hyperventilation in the presence of persistent and uncontrollable pain.' Pain is telling you that you are in danger. We know that changing our breathing in response to pain stimulates the sympathetic side of the nervous system and our body responds to the potential threat or danger of pain. This chapter looks at a few techniques that can be complementary to taking pain medication. They can help by distracting and taking your mind elsewhere or by calming your nervous system, or maybe even by focusing in on the pain to see how it changes and shifts. As always with yoga, there is not a one-size-fits-all, so try some of the different methods to see if one helps more than another.

Pain has two parts: a physical or biological sensation and then a secondary sensation, which is the brain's reaction and the thoughts we apply to that pain. Pain is subjective and our memories and culture will influence the experience. For example, before the experience of cancer you might have ignored a pain but after a diagnosis you might have worrying thoughts about what that pain may imply. Pain can bring up lots of questions as we try to make sense of why we are experiencing it and what that pain may be. Once you have been diagnosed with cancer there is always going to be some fear that it might be cancer causing any pain and our mind can create all kinds of possibilities as to why we are in pain. We want to acknowledge these thoughts but then find some tools to deal with the secondary pain.

As Dean Ornish says in his book *Love and Survival*: 'Pain is a physical process… suffering is the perception of that experience. Even when pain cannot be modified, the experience – suffering – can be greatly reduced.'[5] We will explore some techniques that can help with the perception of pain, like body scans which draw our awareness to other areas of the body and white light meditation that visualises moving pain away from where you feel it.

Studies have shown that yoga helps people cope with physical pain through developing self-discipline (**tapas**) and maintaining a regular practice.[6] So, start small, maybe practising for a minute or so to begin with and then building on that. A shorter but regular practice is better than a long practice every once in a while.

Meditation practices can help us to understand that, although we are in pain, we are not our pain or our thoughts about the pain. You might be identifying with the sensations, but when we close our eyes, we are still the same person inside. Practising self-compassion, like a metta meditation in the chapter on the 'Immune system and infections' (page xx), can help empower you to feel as if you are the driver and not the passenger. Practising non-judgement and helping yourself to accept what is happening and not being hijacked by pain can also provide some ways to cope with the sensations you feel. You could also try some of the eye exercises in the chapter on 'Eyes' (page 81) or the exercises on small movements to release joints in the chapters on 'Joint pain' (page 111) and 'Peripheral neuropathy' (page 193).

Breathing techniques

Focus on natural pauses in the breath

When we are in pain, we often restrict our breathing. Our muscles might contract around the pain, and we might breathe erratically or hold our breath. These breathing patterns send a message to the nervous system that something is wrong and then the body responds to the threat. Our bodies tense up preparing to fight, flee or freeze. Here we want to bring our awareness to our breathing so that it starts to become a bit calmer, deeper or more rhythmic and to see if we can breathe into sensations so that they might soften. Maybe, just maybe, we can actually focus on our pain and not our natural reaction to run away from it, fight it or freeze as a result of it.

Belly breathing

Find a place where you feel safe and supported. It is easier to feel breath into our belly when we are supine (lying down on our spine) as gravity helps us to feel the movement of our breath down into the belly. We want to start to stimulate the parasympathetic side of our nervous system – the 'rest and digest' system. Belly breathing helps to promote a calm, contented state of mind.

Place your hands on your belly or something light over it that allows you to feel it moving up when you breathe in and down when you breathe out. As you start to watch your breathing, can you sense the natural flow in and out? Can you observe that there are some pauses? Inhale and notice that there is a pause and then there is the exhale. After the exhale there is a pause and then your inhale. Can you sense there are gaps?

Focus on the pain

Now bring your awareness to an area where you are experiencing pain. Pain can have a force and amplitude that make it all-consuming, but can you sense that there are also pauses in pain, even if those gaps are tiny micro gaps?

Can you pinpoint the pain to the size of a coin? What happens when you acknowledge the centre of the pain? Does the feeling shift, move, migrate? Does it stay the same or does it throb, pull or pulse? Is it sharp or shooting? Pain, like life, is constantly changing. It can change with your breathing. It is hard to turn towards the pain and observe it and breathe into it when our natural reaction is to want to run away from and avoid pain at all costs. It takes courage and strength to notice the point of pain and to pause, to witness the labels and thoughts we attach to pain and how frightening this can be and observe how we can create more pain or secondary pain by worrying about the pain. What happens to pain when we don't label it as pain? What happens if we stop resisting the pain? Notice your reaction. Can you come back to breathing some warmth into the pain? Can you soften around the point of pain by not trying to block it out but also not reacting to it?

Focus away from pain

Sometimes it may be too intense to focus on the point of pain and you may need to put pain more into the background. If so, can you guide your awareness to an area of your body that is neutral, where there is no pain? Your eyebrows maybe? Know that you have options. You can go elsewhere in your body to areas that aren't in pain and sometimes you may need that avoidance because sometimes it is just too much. If the sensation is too much, rest your attention back on your breathing. Is it changing in response to the pain or your thoughts about the pain? Maybe you find you are holding your breath till the sensations pass? Find those neutral areas of your body. Focus on them and then back to your breath so you can have a break.

Unpleasant sensations trigger thoughts and often fear, and our bodies prepare to fight or flee, so can you use your breath as an anchor to come back to again and again, stimulating the 'rest and reset' response by returning again and again to the rhythm of your breathing like a wave, a wave that massages down through your body? You could also try the point-to-point breathing exercise in the chapter on 'Anxiety and scanxiety' (page 37).

Breath ratios

When we breathe in, we stimulate the sympathetic side of our nervous system and our heart rate speeds up. When we breathe out, we stimulate the soothing parasympathetic side of our nervous system, and our heart rate slows down. You can feel this for yourself. Find your pulse and see what happens when you breathe in and out. Your pulse speeds up when you breathe in, and slows when you breathe out, so your exhale is more calming.

It is widely thought that the optimal breath ratio for pain is 1:2; this would mean breathing in for 1 and out for 2 (in for 2 out for 4, in for 3 out for 6 etc); however, the

quality of breathing is more important than the quantity so find breath ratios that work for you. Try working from the count of your exhale first (rather than the count of your inhale) to find your unique ratio so that breathing doesn't become stressful. Breathe out and count the length of your exhale to find its natural count. Then divide this by two to find your inhale count. Try then breathing in and out to this count and you will have the 1:2 ratio of breathing that suits you.

If this is challenging, try humming with your exhale. This will naturally lengthen it and may be easier to do than counting. Try different sounds and pitches to see if there is a sound that resonates with you, or you feel it vibrating in your body. See vibrational breathing in the chapter on 'Breathing' for more suggestions on sounds (page 49).

Meditations

Body scan

A body scan can build familiarity with your body. Observe the sensations and, if you experience discomfort, notice what does discomfort feel like? If you find it boring, notice what does boredom feel like? Welcome the resistances. Vidyamala Burch and Danny Penman in *Mindfulness for Health*, explain that sometimes a body scan can initially make you feel worse but that this is a good sign.[7] 'As you relax your body has to adjust to the lack of tension and stress. If you have spent years suffering with pain, tension and stress, then it can take years for your body to return to its natural healthy balance of shape and alignment.'

You might practise this body scan from a seated position or from lying down. Make sure you are supported with blankets under your body and head and maybe have something to keep you warm as we often cool down when we come into stillness.

- Bring your awareness down to your toes and sense your toes drifting away from your feet creating space in your feet.
- Soften the soles of your feet, the front of your feet and ankles. Feel the weight of your heels on the floor or mat.
- Soften your calves and feel the weight of your shins resting down onto your calves.
- Feel the front of your knees, the back of your knees. Soften your quadriceps – the muscles at the front of your thighs – and allow the weight of your thighs

to release down into the mat/floor and let your hamstrings soften.

- Soften your groin, and allow all the muscles, tendons and ligaments around your hips to release and feel your legs become heavy and warm as they sink down into the mat/floor.
- Soften your belly, lower back, middle back and upper back. Feel your two shoulder blades making contact with the mat/floor and allow them to soften down into it; as they do so, feel your chest releasing and opening.
- Soften your biceps and triceps, notice the space at your elbows and forearms and the space between your forearms and hands. Rest your awareness in the palms of your hands and then your thumbs, index fingers, middle fingers, ring fingers and little fingers.
- Bring your awareness to the space at the back of your neck and the front of your throat and soften the sides of your throat.
- Release your lower jaw, gums and teeth and allow your tongue to thicken, broaden and soften.
- Let go of your upper jaw, gums and teeth and allow the roof of your mouth to dome upwards towards the crown of your head. Feel your breath gently caressing your nostrils.
- Allow your eyes to soften down into your head and your eyelids to become heavy. Soften the skin across your forehead.
- Feel how you are held by the mat/floor. You don't need to do anything or hold anything; you can just let go. Let go physically. Let go of any thoughts and judgements. If it is hard to settle your mind, have an intention to settle or let go with each exhale.

You can do the body scan on its own or you might want to add a meditation with white light to see if this helps with any pain.

White light meditation

Find a comfortable position, maybe lying down, but if you are more comfortable seated then stay seated.

- Place something light over your belly. This might be your hands or a washcloth or yoga block. Bring your awareness to whatever is placed onto your belly and start to feel it move as you breathe in and out. Feel how it rises as you breathe in and see how it falls as you breathe out.

- Breathe in through your nose and out through your mouth making a sigh or sound to release some tension. Close your mouth if you are okay to breathe in through the mouth; if not, keep it slightly open.
- If you are comfortable, close your eyes, but if not, softly gaze.
- Slowly count your breath as you breathe in.
- Slowly count your breath as you breathe out.
- Stay counting for a few rounds of breathing.
- Bring your awareness to your skin and notice where it makes a connection to the floor, your clothing and the air. Sense that your body is bathed in white light. The white light is nourishing and nurturing.
- As you inhale you start to draw that white light in towards your heart and rest your awareness on your heart. Don't worry about the anatomical placement of your heart but the find the centre of your chest, your energetic heart centre.
- As you inhale white light into your heart, you can say to yourself: 'I am nourished by the light,' or 'I am protected or healed by the light' or find some other positive words or affirmations that might support you right now and have meaning to *you*.
- Sense that your heart starts to become full of light and that you start to visualise a ball of light at your heart and that this ball of light is nourishing, nurturing, protecting and healing and, as you breathe in, you can direct this ball of light to any areas where you are feeling pain. Your inhaled breath is taking healing and nurturing energy to the area of pain.
- As you exhale, your breath draws the ball of light and the pain away from that area.
- Breathing in, your inhale blows the nurturing ball to the pain, easing it.
- Exhale and the ball blows away from the area of pain, taking the pain with it.
- Stay with this sense of the white light nurturing the area that needs tender loving care as you inhale and draws away pain as you exhale.
- You might like to direct the ball of light to other areas of your body or just sense the light pulsing between the place of pain and the release of the pain out of your body.
- Stay with this for as long as you feel comfortable.
- When you are ready to come back and get on with your day, start to deepen your breathing in and out. Bring some movement back into your fingers and toes.

- Stretch out through your body. If you are lying down, roll to one side and press down with your top hand to bring you up to a sitting position.
- Take a moment here to drop your gaze down to your heart and to acknowledge the light or energy that you carry.

Thank you to Nicki Aylwin for sharing this with me.

Scar tissue

Scar tissue is fibrous tissue made up from collagen that replaces the injured skin. It is less elastic and, although it is not sensitive to pain, it can pull on other areas, compress nerves, blood vessels and organs, and can restrict the layers of muscle and connective tissue. It therefore can affect the joints' range of motion and restrict the neural pathways. Even when the size of the external scar looks small, as when lymph nodes are removed, there can be much more scar tissue below the surface. The scar tissue will also vary depending on wound size, depth, location, a person's age and skin colour and this can mean that two separate scars on your body can look very different.

When scar tissue forms after surgery or radiation therapy, there might also be some nerve pain or numbness if the scar tissue forms around nerves. Scar tissue can form in the armpit after lymph nodes have been removed. The connective tissue in the armpit gets inflamed and can form one or more tight bands, known as 'cording'. It is harmless but can be painful and limit movement: the chapter on 'Underarm pain – cording' (page 229) explores stretches that can help to release this tissue.

The lymphatic system does not like scar tissue as this tissue can act like a gate, restricting the flow within and movement of the body. We know that the lymph system relies on movement, so firstly, we want to build back range of motion before starting to build back strength.

Supine poses

Notice how you hold yourself. Even as you read this, do you drop your head forward? Do your shoulders round? Does your lower back round? We do naturally close up the front of our body when we are scared or anxious. It is a way to protect ourselves – we close the front of our body to prevent ourselves getting hurt or to protect our heart from pain. So, a good place to start is by lying supine (on your back) over a rolled-up blanket to open up your chest. You can stay in this restorative 'opening' pose for a few minutes to help to release the tissue and any tension that your body might be holding from treatment or the build-up of scar tissue or from the trauma of surgery.

We have two main chest muscles to open up, the pectoralis ('pec') major and the pectoralis minor.

Stretching the pec minor

The pec minor attaches to the shoulder blade so when it is tight it contributes to the rounding of our shoulders as it pulls the shoulder blade forward. As it is a deeper muscle, the pec minor is harder to stretch than the pec major and takes a bit of time to release.

- Lying over a rolled blanket either running along your spine or across your body underneath your shoulder blades is a good way to get an opening at the front of the body.
- Make sure that the back of your neck feels long. You might need a cushion or blanket under your head.
- You might also like to bend your knees and, if you feel a pulling or tightness in your lower back, try either making the roll smaller or lifting up your bottom and lengthening your tailbone towards your feet and then lowering your bottom back down.
- If the rolled blanket under your shoulder blades feels uncomfortable – and again your breath will become short if it is – then try lying the blanket along the length of your spine. Allow your shoulder blades to drape down towards the floor on either side of it so gravity can help you to open up your chest.
- I find that if I bend my elbows, it allows the opening to be focused on my chest. However, if this movement causes any discomfort then place a folded blanket underneath your arm(s) so that they are supported and therefore can relax. Find an angle with your arm(s) and body that doesn't cause any pain or discomfort and in which you can still breathe smoothly. This is important as, if the pose is uncomfortable, then you won't be able to relax into it and allow the tightly held muscles to release. How we breathe will be affecting our ability to let go so we want to be in a place where we can still breathe in and

out evenly and fluidly.

- You can stay in this position for as long as you feel comfortable, up to 10–15 minutes (see Figure 133).

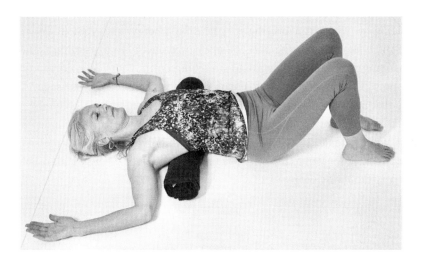

Figure 133: Releasing pec minor

The yoga tradition views the body as an energy field. The *Hatha Yoga Pradipika* speaks of 72,000 nadis or energy channels that carry energy or prana throughout the body.[1] From a western perspective we could view these energy channels as our nervous system carrying information throughout the body. Chinese medicine views these energy channels as meridians. The energy travels through the fascia. So, if the fascia gets damaged, then the energy is no longer able to flow freely. The more we can open up the connective tissue and release areas that feel physically stuck, the better our range of motion will be and the more fluids such as lymph can flow freely, as can prana. Prana is always there but sometimes, when it is restricted, we can feel tired or dull and, by moving the body, we can help the prana, or energy, move around the whole system.

What does your breathing tell you? If you sit or lie down, find your neutral spine and start to observe your breathing, you may notice where you feel breath move in your body. Does your breath move more freely within the front of your body? Can you feel breath move into the sides of your body? Can you feel it in the back of your body? Where do you feel breath? Is it easier to breathe down both sides of your body or does your breath get stuck somewhere? Your breathing will tell you what is going on in your body. Let your breath be your guide. Your breath will highlight areas of tightness. These are areas where your breath gets caught or where it shortens.

Can you sense that the quality of your inhalations is giving, recharging and regenerating so when you breathe in you draw energy into your body with your breath? And when you breathe out, you allow that energy to expand throughout your body? Moving your arms and legs and stretching out in your body, do you find some tighter spots? Can you direct your breath into those areas like a massage? Unlike a massage that applies pressure from the skin on the outside of the body, the massage from your breath comes from the inside as you massage outwards towards your skin.

When you are ready to come out of the pec minor stretch, roll to the side that is most comfortable for you to lie on, move the blanket out of the way and roll back onto your back without any props.

Supine twists

Supine twists give the whole of each side of the body a stretch so you may be aware of pulling or tugging sensations in areas of scar tissue. This can feel intense but should not be painful. Let your breath guide you and, if you find you are holding your breath, ease out of the pose or place blankets on either side of your body to support your legs as you twist.

- Lie on the floor and place your hand behind your head. If this is too much, hold a yoga strap or belt between your two hands behind your head so you aren't in any pain.
- Start with knees bent and feet flat on the floor. Point your elbows up to the ceiling so that your elbows and knees mirror each other.
- **Exhale** and take your knees to the right and open your elbows out and down towards the floor.
- **Inhale** here observing where you are feeling a stretch.
- **Exhale** and bring your knees and elbows back up to point to the ceiling.
- **Inhale**.
- **Exhale** take your knees to the left and open your elbows out and down to the floor (see Figure 134).
- **Inhale** and breathe into any scar intensity.
- **Exhale** and come back to the centre with your knees and elbows.

212

- You can continue moving dynamically from side to side or stay for a few breaths on each side breathing into any areas that feel tight or restricted.

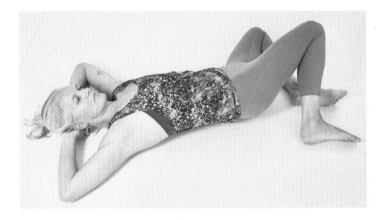

Figure 134: Supine twist: knees over to left

- Then roll to the side that is most comfortable to you, keeping your stronger arm on top so you can use that hand to push into the floor and help yourself to come up to sit. Let your head be the last thing to come up.

Seated poses

With seated poses you want to sit on something that elevates your pelvis higher than your knees, so that you can feel you are on your sitting bones and your lower back travels forward and doesn't become rounded. If you feel that it does then add a few more folded blankets so you are sitting on something higher.

Rib massage

- Taking your left hand to the right side of your ribcage, gently start to massage around the sides of your ribs.
- Move the massage up towards your armpit. Back off if you feel any pain but see if you can release any 'stickiness' you might feel in the connective tissue around your ribcage and armpit area.

213

- Take your left hand to the floor and as you inhale breathe into your ribs and lean to the left, then as you exhale ease out a little bit (see Figure 135).

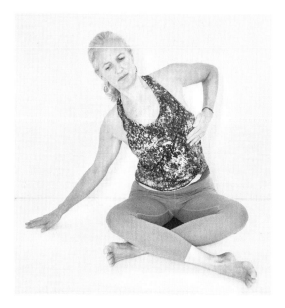

Figure 135: Rib massage – leaning to one side

- Repeat 4–5 times as you inhale, moving into a side stretch whilst massaging your ribs and, when you exhale, ease out of the stretch a bit.
- Sometimes you might find that, with repetition, you can go a little deeper into the pose. You are not forcing yourself into the pose but using your breath to release, let go and move more.
- When you finish the right side, pause.
- Breathe into the two sides of your body and notice if there is more space in one side than the other. Does the side you massaged and breathed into feel more open? Freer? Does the other side feel a bit shorter, denser, or stuck? Observe without judgement.
- Repeat on the left side.

Shoulder blade squeeze

- If you are seated with your legs crossed, change the cross of your legs to create some balance in your pelvis.
- Take your hands behind your back as if putting them into imaginary pockets with palms facing out. Squeeze your shoulder blades together and feel how this opens up your chest (see Figure 136).
- This might feel like enough so you might stay here or interlace your fingers.
- Keep your elbows bent and squeeze your shoulder blades together to open your chest.
- Draw your knuckles away from your body and down without your shoulders rolling forward.
- Check that it doesn't make your head draw forward; take your face back as if you were making a double chin, but not quite that far!

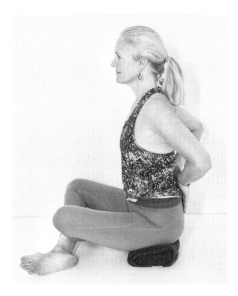

Figure 136: Squeezing shoulder blades together

Seated chest stretch

- Still seated with the top of your pelvis higher than your knees, hold a strap, scarf or belt between your hands and take your hands wide, stretching your arms out in front of you. Pull out on the strap. Doing this helps to relax your upper trapezius and to soften your shoulders down away from your ears. The strap also helps to strengthen you as it engages the muscles of your side waist (obliques) and spine and your large back muscle, the latissimus dorsi.
- Draw your arms back into their sockets and, as you **inhale**, take the strap up towards the ceiling.
- See if you can take your arms up without your ribs poking out into your t-shirt or vest. This will give you an idea of your arm/shoulder mobility and stop you bringing your body into a back bend to get your arms up. The body likes to take the path of least resistance and, if it does, the ribs will move out to help your arms to rise up. Our aim is to eventually have full range of motion but sometimes we have to take baby steps and remember that even little acorns grow into big oak trees. Try not to judge. Try to be kind. Practising kindness *is* yoga.
- As you **exhale**, take the strap behind you until you get a stretch across your chest; you might need to slide your hands along the strap to widen your hand position.
- Pull out against the belt to relax your upper trapezius and allow your shoulders to soften.
- Take a breath in here and a breath out here (see Figure 137). Stay for a few more cycles of breathing if you can.

Chest stretch with bent elbows

Bending your elbows might give you a better or a different stretch across the chest, front of shoulders and arms. If you felt that you got a better stretch with your arms straight, then straighten your arms. Take time to observe what this feels like and take the version that is preferable to you in this moment – the one that gives you the best sense of opening your armpits and chest. Start in the same position as before and again use a long scarf, strap or belt.

- **Inhale** and, holding the scarf, stretch your arms up to the ceiling.
- **Exhale** and pull the belt or strap a little with your left hand, so you lean to the

216

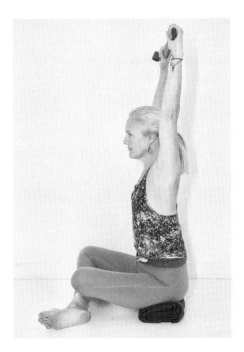

Figure 137: Extending arms to ceiling

left and feel the stretch in your right-side ribs (see Figure 138).

- **Inhale** and move back to the centre.
- **Exhale** and pull a little on the belt or strap with your right hand, so you lean to the right and feel the stretch in your left side (see Figure 139).
- **Inhale** and move back to the centre.
- **Exhale** and lower the strap down. You can put the strap to one side now.
- **Inhale** and take your right elbow up and behind your head. You might feel it towards the middle of your upper back.
- Take your left hand onto your right elbow and press both elbows up. Wrap your right outer arm forward and soften your neck and shoulders (see Figure 140). Your right arm has externally rotated to help open up and release your shoulders.
- You have the option to stay here or to stretch your left arm out in line with your shoulder.

- Turn your thumb down, stretch your arm back, bend your elbow and then take your hand (palm facing out) behind your back; this arm is internally rotated. Try to keep your collarbones broadening so your chest stays open. You might hold onto your t-shirt, or you could hold onto the strap. Keep the left side of your chest opening. This might mean lowering your left hand down towards your lower back (see Figure 141).
- Take a few breaths here and, when you release, roll your shoulders or take your fingers to your shoulders and make circles with your elbows 6 times in one direction and 6 times in the other.
- Change sides, taking your left elbow up.

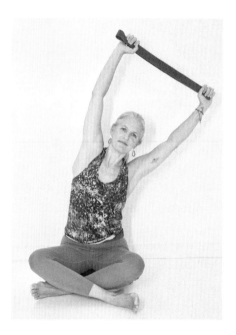

Figure 138: Stretching to the left

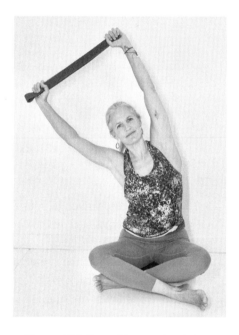

Figure 139: Stretching to the right

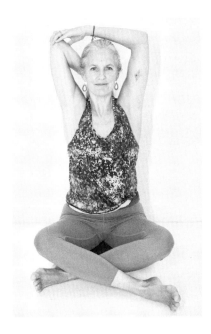

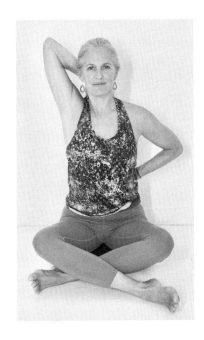

Figure 140: Taking elbows up and back above head

Figure 141: Left arm dropping down behind back

Puppy pose

- Come onto all fours. You might need a blanket under your knees for padding. The puppy pose is a good pose for stretching the arms, armpits and sides of the ribs.
- Bring your elbows to the floor. If you can, keep them touching as you drop your face to rest your cheeks between your arms (see Figure 142).

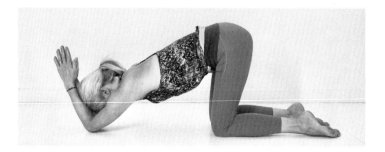

Figure 142: Puppy pose on elbows

- Walk your knees back so you can create some traction and lengthening along your spine, and you feel a stretch.
- Try not to let your lower back collapse by drawing your ribs and belly away from the floor. This might feel like you are toning your belly. This should support your lower back, stop you feeling the stretch there and help to focus the stretch in your upper body. It can be intense, but it shouldn't be painful.

Standing postures

Dynamic trikonasana

- Take hold of your strap or belt with both hands.
- Step your feet wide apart. Your feet should be in line with each other.
- Turn your right toes out 90°. Pick up your left heel and turn it slightly out.
- Press down evenly with both feet so you feel equal weight in both.
- Press into the ball of your right (now front) foot. Engage the front of your thigh – your quadriceps; this will work to lift your kneecap and you will feel the front of your leg firm without locking out. Your leg will look straight but you will be able to feel that it isn't locked straight and has a little microbend in it.
- Hold the strap wider than shoulder-distance apart and pull out on it so that it is taut.
- **Inhale** and take the strap up. Pull out on it (see Figure 143).
- **Exhale** and drop the right side of your bottom down and back towards your left heel.

- Keeping length through the right side of your spine, your pelvis will shift to the left as you come into this modified trikonasana. Keep a micro-bend in your front rightknee (it looks straight but you know it isn't fully straight) so that you are hinging at the hips and there isn't any pressure at the knee (see Figure 144).
- Press down through your feet and **inhale**, then use your legs, not your lower back, to bring you up to standing (see Figure 143).
- **Exhale** and lower the strap down (see Figure 145).
- Repeat 4 more times.
- You will feel that your core is working here to support your body, stopping your torso collapsing over the right leg and your spine from rounding, and helping to build some strength in the sides of your body, as well as stretching the left side of your ribs.
- Repeat on the left side.
- Step your feet back together and shake out your legs to release any tension.

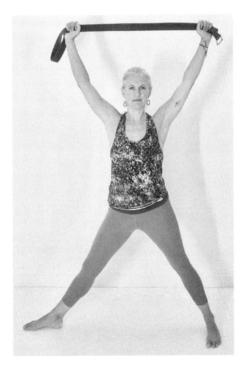

Figure 143: Pulling out on strap

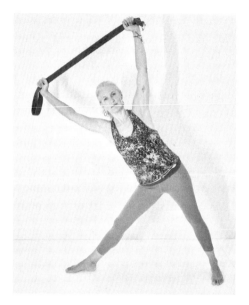

Figure 144: Hinging at hips without pressure on knee

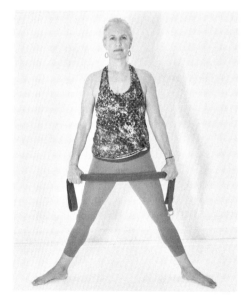

Figure 145: Lowering strap

Dynamic horse stance

- Step your feet wide apart. Your feet should be in line with each other. The wider, the more challenging so you can always bring your feet closer together to make it a little easier.
- Turn the toes of both feet out. Your knees should be going in the same direction as your toes.
- Take your hands wide on the strap or scarf. If you want more of a challenge, then you could bring your hands a little closer together.
- **Inhale**, take the strap up and bend your knees and elbows into a goal-post shape (see Figure 146).
- **Exhale**, bend your elbows and turn to the right (see Figure 147).
- **Inhale**, come back to the centre and reach your arms to the ceiling (see Figure 148).
- **Exhale** and bend you elbows and turn to the left (see Figure 149).
- **Inhale**, turn back to the centre and reach your arms towards the ceiling.
- **Exhale**, lower the strap and straighten your legs.
- Repeat as often as you have energy for (4–8 times).

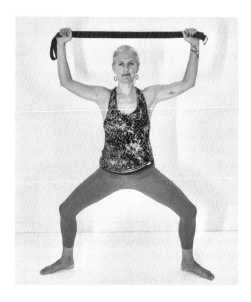

Figure 146: Taking strap up and bending elbows and knees

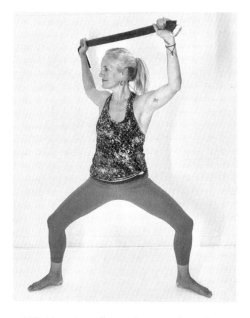

Figure 147: Keeping elbows bent and turning to right

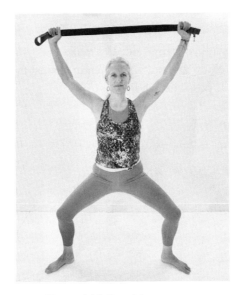

Figure 148: Reaching arms up

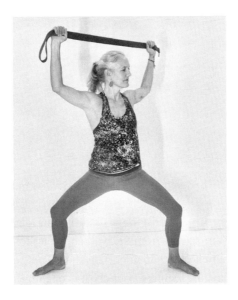

Figure 149: Bending elbows and turning to left

Wall chest stretches

- Stand sideways with your right side to a wall.
- Bend your right elbow and put your forearm against the wall as close to shoulder height as possible (see Figure 150).

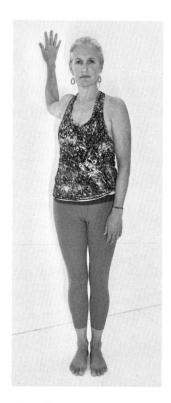

Figure 150: Bending elbow and putting forearm against wall

- Keeping your forearm against the wall, turn your toes away from the wall so that your body turns away from the wall and you feel a gentle stretch on the right side of your chest or shoulder. You should not feel pain, but it may feel intense, or it may just feel like your chest is opening.
- Breathe into your chest, armpit and shoulder. Stay here for eight breaths, turning your gaze away from the wall.
- To release, turn back to the wall.

- Lower your right arm down and close your eyes to observe what it feels like. Notice the height of your two shoulders, notice if your arms feel the same length or if one feels longer and sense any sensations in your arm, chest or shoulder. Does any area of your body feel more awake or alive?

Bridge lifts

Bridge lifts can be a good way to lengthen and stretch along the front of the body and release tension held in the belly.

- Lie on your back on a mat without any blankets or cushions under your head as this can flatten the lovely curve in your neck as you start to move.
- Lift your hips away from the floor.
- Lengthen your knees away from your head.
- Lengthen your pubic bones and tailbone towards your knees to facilitate more stretch in the front of your body.
- You can continue moving with your breath, inhaling to lift your hips and exhaling to lower them, or stay in this position for a few breaths.
- If you need more support, you could place a brick or bolster under your pelvis so the stretch becomes a passive as opposed to an active stretch (see Figure 151).

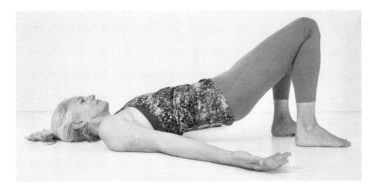

Figure 151: Bridge lift

To finish

- To finish, try the **releasing pec minor** with blanket (page 211) or lying over a bolster or blanket lengthways along the spine to see if this feels like it opens your chest in a kinder way than the blanket running under your shoulder blades. Take the pose that works best for you.
- You could also finish in a **supta baddha konasana** to open the front of your chest, belly and pelvis (see Figure 38 in the chapter 'Digestive problems and discomfort', page 76).
- Breathe in fully.
- Breathe out fully.

Underarm pain – cording

Pain may be due to cord-like structures that can form as part of scar tissue and are harmless but can limit arm movement and be painful. This cording may be just in the armpit or may extend down the arm to the hand or across to the chest. Often known as 'axillary web syndrome', they are thought to be due to inflammation and scarring of tissues that surround the lymph vessels, blood vessels and nerves. The following sequences aim to stretch into the armpit and arm while at the same time avoiding anything that causes pain. The stretching can feel intense, and you may get a popping sensation as sometimes the cords snap. This is nothing to worry about and should feel like a good release after the pop.

Supine poses

Supine chest opener

- Start by lying on your back over a bolster or blanket to open up your chest.
- Stay in this position for up to 5 minutes. Start with your arms out in line with your shoulders, palms facing up, bending your elbows and supporting the backs of your hands on the blankets if they are unable to rest comfortably on the floor.
- There shouldn't be any pain, but it might feel intense across your chest, shoulders and arms. There may be a difference on one side; this is totally natural (see Figure 152).
- If this feels too much, then come off the bolster or blanket and make it smaller.

- If you feel discomfort in your lower back, press your feet into the floor or mat, lift your bottom away from the floor and lengthen your tailbone away from your head so it feels like your spine lengthens; then lower your bottom back down.
- If you still feel discomfort in your lower back, make the bolster or blanket smaller again.

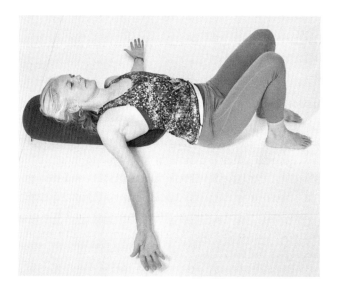

Figure 152: Supine chest opener alternative to Figure 133

Snow angels

- Lie on your back.
- Slowly, and in increments, start to slide your arms away from your body along the floor towards your ears.
- You will start to feel a greater stretch or opening but try not to push into anything that feels like pain.
- Your breathing will tell you if you have gone too far – for example, if you notice that you have stopped breathing and are holding your breath, waiting for the exercise to be over! If your breathing becomes more erratic and it feels like speed bumps have appeared in it, then find a position for your arms

where you can still breathe in and out fully, ironing out those speed bumps.

- Then start moving dynamically.
- **Exhale** and take your arms down by your sides with your palms facing up.
- **Inhale** and start to slide your hands along the floor towards your ears again.
- **Exhale** and lower your arms back down.
- Don't push into pain but find the angle of your arms where you start to feel a stretch. Try bending your elbows if it feels too much with your arm straight. For more of a challenge you could hover your hands away from the floor as you make 'snow angels'.

Shoulder circles

- Then, bend your elbows and bring your fingertips to your shoulders. Start to circle your shoulders in one direction 6 times and then change direction for another 6 circles.
- Roll off the blanket and come to lie on the mat with your knees bent.

Internally/externally rotating arms

- Then, take your arms up so they are in line with your shoulders (like a capital T) and turn your palms down.
- Then turn your palms up, so you internally and externally rotate your arms. Explore your range of motion here as you repeat this movement 5–8 times.
- Then slide your arms back down alongside your body.

Supine twists

- To increase the stretch on the right side of your body, drop your knees over to the left and then slide your right arm up towards your ears until you feel a stretch in your chest or armpit. Take five breaths here.
- **Exhale**, bring your knees up and lower your right arm down.
- Repeat on the other side and **exhale**, turning your knees to the right and sliding your left arm up towards your ear.
- You may want to repeat these moves a few times on each side holding the twist for five breaths. If this feels too much, or you feel discomfort in your lower back, try putting a cushion between your thighs or underneath the leg

that is closest to the floor.

- To create more stretch in your chest and arms, use your hand to create a gentle tractioning of your skin to release tight tissue and cording.
- As your knees go to the left, reach out through your right arm and use your left hand to gently pull in the opposite direction to your right arm.
- If your twist was to the right, then you would reach out through your left arm and use your right hand to create some traction away from your left wrist (see Figure 153).

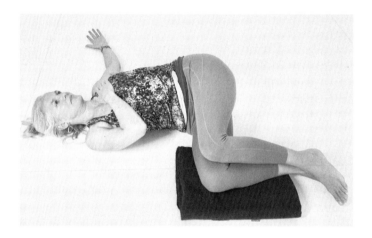

Figure 153: Creating traction with hand in supine twist

- Roll onto your back. Reach your arms up to the ceiling and interlace your fingers. Feel the back of your ribcage on the mat and keep your ribcage drawing down towards the floor.
- **Inhale** and stretch your arms towards your ears, trying to straighten your elbows.
- **Exhale** and bring your arms up towards the ceiling.
- **Inhale** and stretch your arms back towards your ears, keeping your ribs drawn in.
- **Exhale** and bring your arms back up, pointing towards the ceiling.
- Release your interlaced fingers and stretch them up towards the ceiling; squeeze your shoulder blades as you pull your shoulder heads towards the

floor (arms come back into their sockets but elbows stay straight).

- Then broaden your shoulder blades away from your spine and reach your arms up to the ceiling, with your elbows staying straight. Continue a few more times protracting and retracting your shoulder blades as they come towards and away from your spine.

Kneeling poses

Dynamic all fours

- Lie on your back on your mat.
- Then, rolling to the side that you are most comfortable on, press down with your top (stronger arm) to come up onto all fours.
- From all fours **inhale**.
- **Exhale** and drop your bottom back towards your heels.
- **Inhale** and come back up to all fours.
- **Exhale**, drop your bottom back down towards your heels again and inch your fingers a little further forward each time (this is the Child's pose, see Figure 91, page 147). If this feels too much, then bend your elbows towards the floor as you drop your bottom back.
- If you want more of a stretch, straighten your elbows and inch fingers further forward.
- Repeat 3–4 more times.

Because the aim of this is to stretch out under the armpits and arms try to feel that you are lengthening away from your hands and don't worry if your bottom doesn't come back to your heels. If the flexion at your knees or hips feels uncomfortable, walk your hands further forward so when you draw back towards your heels you still feel your armpits opening.

Child's pose with arm stretch

- Go on to all fours again and take your right hand off to the left. (If you are using a mat, it may come off the edge.) Then walk your right hand to meet your left. You may even be able to place your right hand on top of your left but if this feels too intense then keep them alongside each other.

- **Inhale** and then, as you **exhale**, drop your ears in line with your arms as you draw your bottom back towards your heels.
- **Inhale** and come back up to all fours, keeping your hands to the left (see Figure 154).
- **Exhale** and keep your ears in line with your arms and bottom as you sink back towards your heels (see Figure 155).
- Repeat 3 more times.
- Walk your hands back to the centre; then take your right hand out to the right and your left hand right to meet your right hand, repeating on the right side.
- Walk your hands back towards your knees and come to a high kneeling position.
- Hook your thumbs together and rest them on top of your head (see Figure 156). **Inhale** and press your thumbs up towards the ceiling (see Figure 157).
- **Exhale** and lower your arms back to the top of your head.
- Re-bend your elbows and rest your hands on your head. **Inhale** and press your thumbs towards the ceiling, starting to straighten your arms; then **exhale** and lower your hands back towards your head.
- Repeat a few more times, not pushing into pain but sensing any intensity and breathing into it.
- Release out of the pose and come to stand.

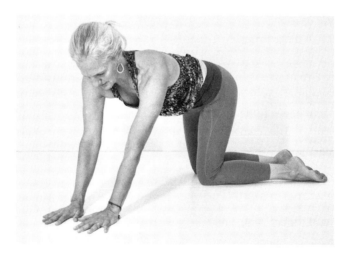

Figure 154: Hands to the left on all fours

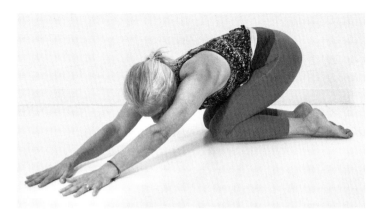

Figure 155: Hands to the left moving back into child's pose

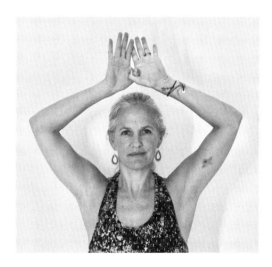

Figure 156: Thumbs locked, elbows bent, hands on head

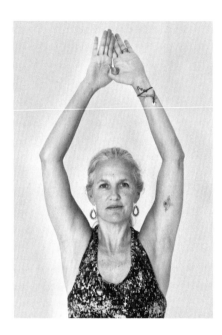

Figure 157: Thumbs locked, arms straight and extending up

Dynamic child's pose with asymmetrical arms

- From all fours slide your right hand forward, keeping your left hand where it is (see Figure 158). You can elevate your right hand with a yoga block, but if when you move this feels too intense, take your hand back to the floor and move through the sequence without a block. Tone your belly and breathe into the back of your ribcage so your ribs don't poke out at the front of your body, and you don't collapse down into your shoulder socket. Move in a pain-free way.
- **Inhale** here.
- **Exhale** whilst lowering your bottom towards your heels (you can always place a blanket on your calves if you feel this in your knees – the blanket just helps to keep some space at the back of the knee) and bending your left elbow. Keep pressing down through your right hand (see Figure 159).
- **Inhale** and move back to all fours; **exhale** and lower your bottom towards your heels.
- Repeat 4 more times.

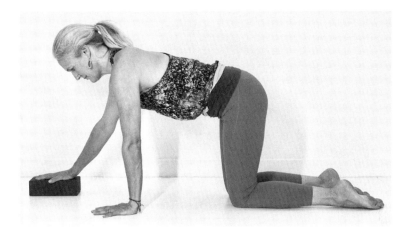

Figure 158: Sliding right hand forward whilst kneeling

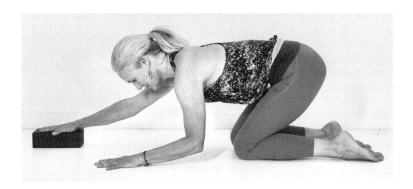

Figure 159: Bending left elbow whilst lowering bottom

- Come back to all fours and slide your right hand under your left arm to come into a twist. Reach with your right arm along the floor to the left (see Figure 160).

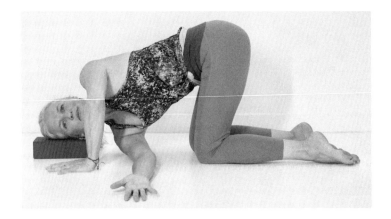

Figure 160: Sideways twist reaching with right hand to the left

- Bring either the side of your head or your cheek down to the floor or on to a yoga brick, so you are gazing under your left arm. If this feels too much or causes you any pain, come up to sitting and cross your right arm across your body.
- Breathe into your right shoulder blade for 4–5 breaths.
- Press your left hand into the floor or mat and come up to all fours.
- Change sides, sliding your left hand forward under your right arm.
- Repeat on both sides.
- Release out of the pose and come to standing.

Standing poses

Dynamic warrior II

- Step your feet wide and face the long edge of your mat if you are using one. Check your heels are in line with each other
- Turn your right toes out 90° and pick up your left heel and turn it slightly out. Press down through both feet and feel that there is even weight in both. Keep that as you start to bend your right knee so that your right knee is in line with your right ankle. Just check that the knee doesn't go beyond the ankle, so you are not putting too much pressure on the kneecap (patella).
- Take your hands to the back of your head and press your elbows out wide.

You can always hold a belt if it is challenging to take your hands to the back of your head.

- Check your ribs don't poke out into your t-shirt. Breathe into the back of your body to lift your back ribs out of your lower back (see Figure 161).
- **Inhale**.
- **Exhale** and squeeze your elbows towards each other as you straighten your right leg (see Figure 162).
- **Inhale**, bend your right knee and press your elbows out, away from each other.
- **Exhale**, straighten your right leg and squeeze your elbows towards each other.
- Repeat 3 more times.
- Then, bending your front (right) knee, **exhale**, firming your belly and leaning to the right, in a modified side angle pose (see Figure 163).

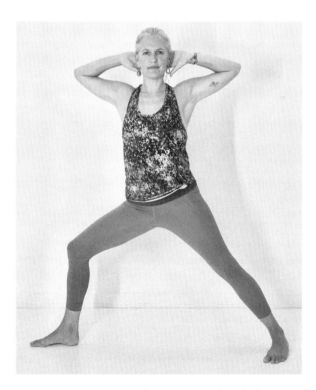

Figure 161: Warrior II with hands on head and elbows wide

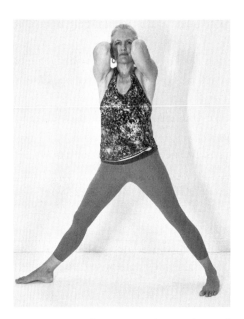

Figure 162: Squeeze elbows together and straighten leg

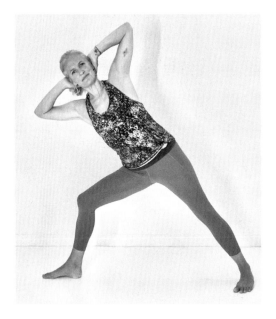

Figure 163: Modified side-angle pose

Side-angle pose

- Lower either your right hand or your right forearm to your right thigh. Press down with your hand or forearm so you don't collapse onto the leg.
- Lift your side waist away from your right leg.
- Circle the top (left) arm with the elbow bent (see Figure 164), with the option to start to straighten this arm if there is no impingement in your shoulder.
- Sweep your left elbow/arm a little bit behind you as you circle it so that you open up your chest, but back off if you feel discomfort in the shoulder joint.
- Keep your ribs softening down towards your hips and draw your pubic bone towards your belly button to firm your belly and support your lower back.

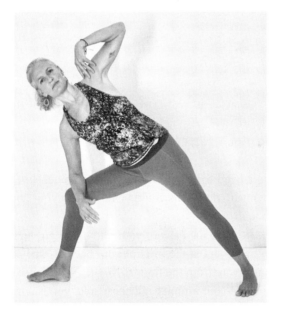

Figure 164: Side-angle pose with circling elbow

Chair down dog

- Bend your knees so that you can forward fold at the top of your thighs and keep your spine long as you bring your hands down to hold onto the sides of the seat of a chair (see Figure 165).

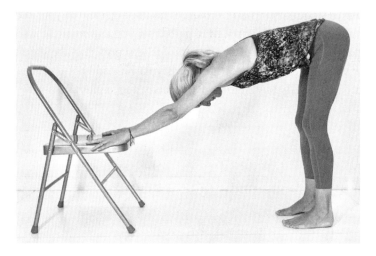

Figure 165: Chair-assisted downward dog

- Then, keeping a bend in your knees and a long spine, start to walk your feet back into downward dog. This could be done with your hands on a wall instead of a chair.
- Bring more breath into the back of your body, filling it with breath so that your ribs don't poke out at the front of your body. Tone your belly and suck your armpits up away from the floor so you don't collapse in your shoulders.
- If this is intense on your armpits and chest area, you can move in and out of the pose dynamically with your breathing. Shift forward with your shoulders as you inhale and then press your inner thighs back to come back into the stretch as you exhale.
- Take 5–6 dynamic breaths or stay static, then step your right foot forwards towards the chair, bend your left knee and bring the knee to the mat or floor; then step your right knee back to come to high kneeling.

Puppy pose on chair

- From a high kneeling position, bring your elbows to rest on the seat of the chair. If comfortable, bring in your elbows together so they touch, and draw your bottom back to rest your face in between your arms.
- To increase the stretch, walk your knees back away from the chair.
- To decrease the stretch, walk them closer to the chair.
- This should give you a stretch along your arms, armpits and upper back. To prevent collapsing into your lower back, tone your belly, draw your front ribs in and breathe into the back of your body.
- If this feels too much, then bring your elbows onto the mat or floor instead of the chair (see Figure 142, page 220).

Side-lying poses

These side-lying poses are only suitable if you can comfortably lie on your side. If you can't, you could do a supine twist instead as described at the beginning of this chapter (page 23).

Protraction and retraction of shoulder blades

- To try to get more stretch into your chest, lie on your right side. Use blankets under your head and maybe blankets under your ribs to make it more comfortable to lie on your side.
- Stretch your right arm out in front of your body with your left arm on top.
- Slide your top (left) hand over your bottom (right) hand towards your body as you draw your top arm back into the shoulder socket (retracting the shoulder blade).
- Then start to stroke back along your right arm until you come back to your starting position and the shoulder blade moves away from your spine ('protracting' the shoulder blade).
- Repeat 4–5 times. Try to limit any rocking of your body so it is just your top (left) arm moving forward and back (see Figure 166).

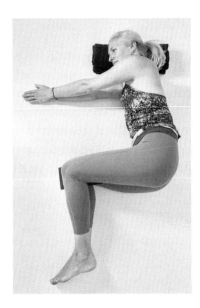

Figure 166: Protracting and retracting shoulder blades

Chest opening into twist

- Remain lying on your right side and continue to stroke your left arm along your right arm.
- Then start to take your left arm across your chest, continuing to open your left arm out to the left, and then slide your left arm back to rest on top of the right.
- Continue with this movement, maybe starting to open your chest towards the ceiling and, as you do, allow your body to move with you as you start to open your chest and your gaze towards the ceiling. You can roll across the back of your head rather than picking up your head to turn it from gazing to the right to gazing towards the ceiling.
- Take your time to come in and out of the pose, maybe going a little further into the twist each time. If you find tight areas, pause, hold them and breathe into them so you use your breath like a massage to open up your body from the inside out (see Figure 167).

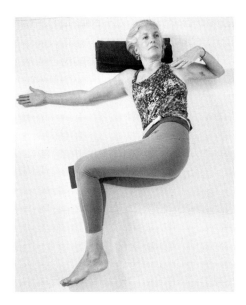

Figure 167: Chest opening into a twist

- Once you feel comfortable with opening into a twist, you could start to add on circling your arm. This is quite a big movement so you might prefer to start with your elbow bent. Bring your left hand to your left shoulder and start to draw a circle with your left elbow. You could continue to keep your left elbow bent or start to straighten it out and circle your arm.
- Repeat lying on your left side.

To finish

- Finish with the supine chest opener described at the beginning of the chapter (page 209) to release and open up through your chest and arms. Hold for 3–5 minutes to release tissue at the front of your body.
- Alternatively, you could finish by lying (supine) over a rolled-up blanket that you have placed under your shoulder blades, with your arms over the roll and your head resting on the floor or on another folded blanket. You may find that you prefer one of these chest openers more or that one gives you a better

opening than the other (see Figure 133, page 211).

- You can stretch out through your arms or bend your elbows so that you experience an opening at the front of your body but no pain. You can always make the blanket roll smaller if it feels like too much. You might be more comfortable with your knees bent or prefer to straighten your legs.
- Breathe in.
- Breathe out.
- Continue consciously breathing in and breathing out.

Weakness in muscles – building strength

Muscle mass is lost during chemo and surgery and weakness can cause problems with balance as well as increasing feelings of fatigue. We often think of yoga as being all about relaxation, but active exercise is beneficial as it strengthens muscles and bones and can provide a sense of empowerment. We lose between 3 and 8% of muscle mass every decade after the age of 30[1] and, as our bodies are designed to move, periods of bed rest or inactivity can cause muscles to atrophy. It is estimated that almost 50% of muscle strength is lost after 3-5 weeks of bed rest.[2, 3] Whilst going through treatment we want to try to minimise muscle loss and, after treatment we want to start to build back muscle strength. Breastcancer.org cite two small studies that suggest that women with more muscle mass are more likely to have milder chemotheraphy side effects than women with less muscle mass.[4]

Loss of muscle strength and range of motion can make standing poses more challenging but the more that we can build back strength in the muscles, the easier it will be to do normal everyday activities like climbing stairs. A huge side effect is often fatigue; this may make you not want to exercise but the more we build strength then the less fatigued we will be in our daily life.

Building strength in muscles will also help with confidence as feeling stronger empowers us to be able to do the normal things we like to do, whatever they might be – walking the dog, taking the kids to school or carrying shopping home from the supermarket. This increases our quality of life, because quality of life is based around being able to perform daily activities without pain or discomfort. If we can strengthen our muscles and learn how to activate muscles around joints, this can help reduce joint pain as muscles take up some of the weight and pressure so that joints are not doing all the work themselves. Muscle strength also increases bone density as the muscle pulls on bone and stimulates more bone tissue.

When we come into active yoga poses, our muscles contract to come in and out of the pose as well as to hold it. We move dynamically in yoga for cancer so that the muscles get strengthened throughout a larger range of motion; muscles get longer whilst relaxing and then shorter whilst contracting. Your muscles work differently when you hold a pose as they get strengthened through isometric muscle contraction (the muscle is firming but not changing length).

If you find any of the standing poses too much, you can modify them using a wall or chair. Use your breathing to stay present and mindful with your movements and gaze at the horizon to help with balance.

If you have metastatic bone cancer, then exercising safely is really important. According to Macmillan Cancer Support: 'A lack of activity leads to muscle atrophy, which can, in fact, increase the likelihood of skeletal complications such as fracture and bone pain.'[5] If you experience any of the red flags, such as bone pain in vertebrae that is worse at night, bone pain in the thigh bone (femur) with weight-bearing poses or a worsening bone pain, then you need to seek medical advice. See the chapter on 'Osteoporosis' (page 171) for advice on moving the spine in a safe way.

Warm-up sequence

Start with the warm-up sequence described at the beginning of the book (Figures 1 to 16, pages 19–29).

Supine poses

Bridge lifts

- If you have a blanket under your head, remove it and place it to one side. Bend your knees, with your feet hip-distance apart and press your feet evenly into the floor.
- Feel your feet and notice that if you roll to their outer edges your knees move outwards and if you roll to their inner edges your knees knock in. Press evenly through your feet so that your knees stay pointing to the ceiling and don't roll in or out.

- You can also place a yoga block between your thighs and gently hold it there to keep your legs active and your feet pressing down evenly into the floor or mat.
- **Inhale** and lift your hips away from the floor like an elevator (see Figure 151, page 227).
- **Exhale** and lower your hips back down.
- **Inhale**, lift your hips again and pause. Can you feel your bottom muscles (glutes) working? You can feel with your hands if your glutes are working to lift up. One may be working more than the other. Firm them without squeezing or clenching; Doug Keller, my anatomy teacher, would say 'think firm like a grape and not wrinkled like a raisin'.
- Then continue moving your hips up and down in time with your breathing 4–5 more times.
- If this feels challenging, you can start with a yoga brick on the floor under your pelvis; lift your pelvis away from the brick and then lower it back down onto the brick.
- If you want more of a challenge, lower your pelvis down but don't touch it to the floor or rest before you lift it back up.

Bridge lifts on heels

- Then walk your feet a little bit away from your bottom and lift the balls of your feet away from the floor; pressing down into your heels, lift your hips, then **exhale** and lower back down (see Figure 168).
- Repeat 3–4 more times, maybe building up to 10–15 repetitions, moving with your breathing.

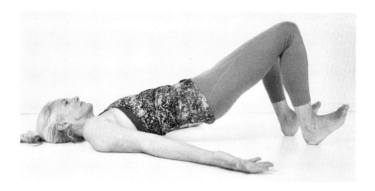

Figure 168: Bridge lift on heels

Figure-of-four

- You can stretch out your glutes into a figure-of-four.
- Cross your right ankle over your left knee and, as you **exhale**, draw your left knee towards you.
- You can hold onto the back of your left leg or elevate your left foot on to a block.
- Breathe in and breathe out.
- Try tipping slightly to the left to see if you can feel different muscle fibres getting a stretch (see Figure 11 in the warm-up exercises in the Introduction, page 25).
- Repeat on the left side.
- Roll over to the side most comfortable to you. Press down with your top hand and, with your head coming up last, come up to all fours.

Kneeling poses

Scapula press ups

- Come onto all fours and bring your forearms to the floor. Keep them in line with your shoulders. (If you are not sure, catch hold of opposite elbows with opposite hands to measure the distance then release your forearms back to the mat or floor.)
- Allow your chest to drop towards the floor. Feel your shoulder blades coming towards each other (see Figure 169).
- As you **exhale**, press your chest away from the floor and feel your shoulder blades drawing away from your spine (see Figure 170).
- Repeat 5–8 more times, starting to activate the muscles between your shoulder blades. Try not to move your head up and down or your lower back but just your upper back so you get to strengthen the muscles that support your shoulder blades.
- Sit your bottom back towards your heels to rest your arms or come to a high kneel and circle your wrists in one direction a few times and then change and circle them the other way.

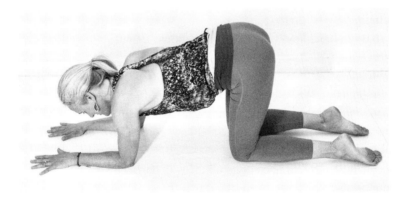

Figure 169: Scapula press up – shoulder blades together

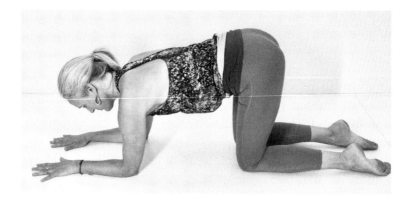

Figure 170: Scapula press up – shoulder blades apart

Transition using core

- Come back to all fours and place your hands on blocks to elevate the floor. Push the floor away from you so you know you are not collapsing down between your shoulder blades and your back feels broad. Lightly tone your belly so you don't collapse down into your lower back and your back feels flat.
- Slide your left leg back keeping the tone of your belly and not collapsing down into your lower back. Your left side is in a half plank (see Figure 171).
- **Inhale**.
- **Exhale** and feel how your belly tones, draws in and slightly up towards your heart.
- **Inhale**.
- **Exhale**, tone your belly and step your left foot forward in between your hands for the lunge. (If you want 'more core' then you can repeat this a few more times using the exhale and your core to help you step your foot forward.)
- If you find your foot doesn't go all the way between your hands, you can use your hands to help lift it and step it forward (see Figure 172).

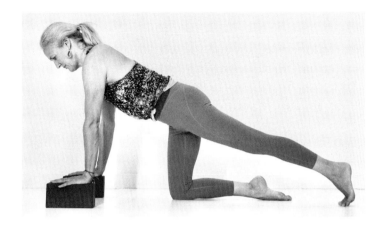

Figure 171: Half plank transition with left leg back

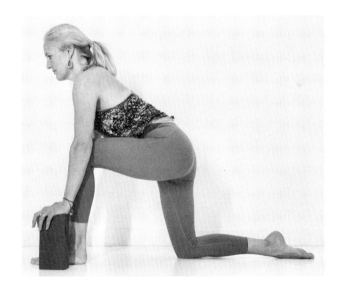

Figure 172: Lunge with back knee down on floor

Lunge

- Raise the blocks to a height where you feel that your spine stays in neutral and doesn't round. Then, tucking your back (right) toes under, lift your back (right) knee away from the mat or floor (see Figure 173).
- **Inhale** here, and then, as you **exhale**, bend your right knee almost to the floor as you press out through your back (right) heel (see Figure 174).
- **Inhale** and lift your right knee back up and **exhale**, lowering it almost to the floor. Continue 3 more times.
- Then lower your right knee to the mat or floor and bring your left knee back so you come back to all fours, keeping your hands on the blocks.
- Repeat on the opposite side.

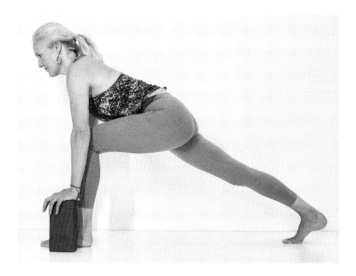

Figure 173: Lunge with back knee lifted

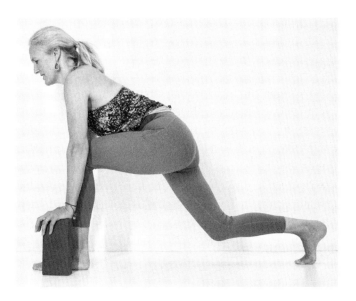

Figure 174: Lunge lowering back knee nearly to the floor

Chair pose

- From the lunge, step your back foot forward to join your front foot and bend both knees as if you were sitting back into an imaginary chair or, if this is too low for you, then back on to an imaginary bar stool.
- Press your forearms to your thighs to keep your back long (see Figure 115, page 179).
- Take a few breaths here.
- The quadriceps (large muscle at the front of the thigh) will be working here.
- Push your bottom back as you stretch your chest forward and if you press into your heels, you should feel your glutes (buttock muscles) working. Try to get the muscles at the front and back of your body working evenly.
- Press down through your feet and come up to stand.

Standing poses

Dynamic warrior II

- Step your feet wide and face the long edge of your mat if you are using one. Check your heels are in line with each other.
- Turn your left toes out 90° and pick up your right heel, turning it slightly out. Press down through both feet and feel that there is even weight in them both. Keep that as you start to bend your left knee so that your right knee is in line with your right ankle. Just check that the knee doesn't go beyond the ankle, so you are not putting too much pressure on your kneecap (patella).
- **Inhale** bringing your arms in line with your shoulders (see Figure 175).
- **Exhale** and straighten the front (left) leg and lower your arms down (see Figure 176).

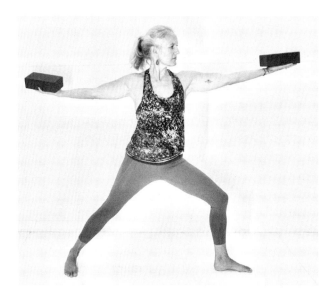

Figure 175: Warrior II, with block option

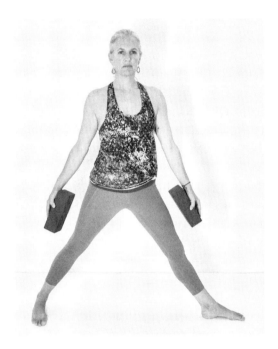

Figure 176: Straightening front leg and lowering arms

- **Inhale** and come back into warrior II, with your arms in line with your
  shoulders and **exhale**, straightening your front (left) leg and lowering your
  arms back down.
- Repeat a few more times, preparing your body to come into warrior II and
  stay. Press down evenly through both feet. Check your front (left) knee isn't
  rolling in towards your big toe. If you think it is, you can lift your left heel
  and then stretch out from your inner thigh to your inner (left) knee and guide
  the knee towards your middle toes.
- Hold for five breaths then press down through your feet to straighten your
  legs, lower your arms and turn to the right to repeat on the right side.
- You can also use the option of holding yoga bricks in your hands as you do
  this pose, as shown in Figures 175 and 176, to make it more challenging and
  help to gain more strength in your arms as you move in and out of warrior II.
  You could also use anything you have at home to add more weight to your
  arms, be it cans of soup or small hand-held weights.

Dynamic heel lifts with chair and yoga brick

- Step to the front of the mat if using.
- Take a yoga brick between your thighs, finding the width of block that feels most comfortable. Gently hug the block with your thighs so you feel the muscles pulling in towards the bone. Also notice your feet: can you feel evenly between the little-toe side of your foot and the big-toe side? Press your feet slightly away from each other so that your outer and inner thighs work evenly.
- **Inhale**, lift your heels and float your arms in front of you and up towards the ceiling. You could also interlace your fingers to support an arm with a limited range of motion if this is an issue for you (see Figure 121, page 186).
- **Exhale** and lower your heels and arms. Bend your knees as if you are sitting back into an imaginary chair (see Figure 122, page 187).
- **Inhale** and float your arms up.
- **Exhale** and sit a bit deeper.
- **Inhale** and straighten your legs to come up to standing. You could also lift your heels as you come up to stand.
- **Exhale** and lower your heels and arms.
- Repeat 5 more times and then release the block from between your thighs.
- You can also try repeating the pose but move slowly as you lower your arms back down so the muscle contracts and lengthens at the same time. To make it more challenging you could repeat the pose but hold a second block between your hands, pressing the palms of your hands flat to the sides of the block to activate the muscles of your arms. Check your ribs don't poke out into your clothing as you take your arms up.

Side bend with brick

- Keep the yoga brick between your thighs and for more challenge hold a second brick or paperback book between your hands. If this feels too much, then let go of the brick or book.
- **Inhale** and raise your arms (see Figure 177).
- **Exhale** and reach up and over to the left (see Figure 178).
- **Inhale** and move back to the centre.
- **Exhale** and reach up and over to the right (see Figure 179).

- **Inhale** and move back to the centre.
- **Exhale** and lower your arms.
- Repeat 2 more times. If it is too much with the block in your hands, then get rid of it. We want to build back muscle strength slowly so if it is too much, do the same sequence but without the block.
- Then release the block from between your thighs.

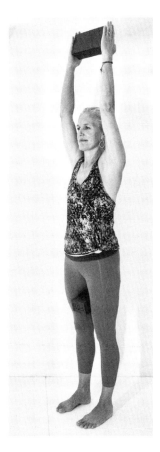

Figure 177: Raising arms with yoga brick

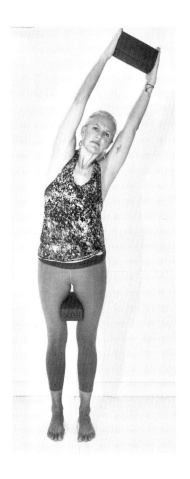
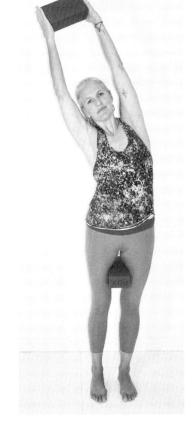

Figure 178: Reaching over to left holding yoga brick

Figure 179: Reaching over to right holding yoga brick

Core climbing

It can be useful to recruit our core when walking upstairs so that not all the work is in our legs.

- Stand with your feet hip-distance apart and your hands on your belly.
- **Inhale** and feel your breath move down into your body.
- **Exhale**: can you sense that your belly draws in and slightly up?
- Repeat a few more times. When we exhale our diaphragm and pelvic floor draw up towards our heart. We want to use this internal lift to help us lift our legs.
- **Inhale** and raise your arms forward and up (see Figure 180).
- **Exhale** and notice how your belly draws in and up as you lower your arms and lift your left foot away from the floor (see Figure 181).

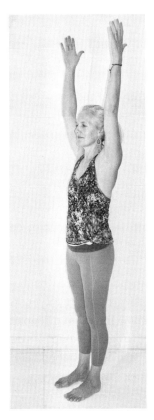

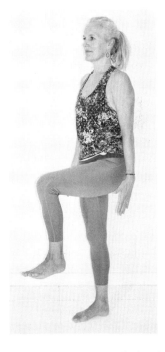

Figure 181: Lowering arms, balancing on right foot, lifting left foot

Figure 180: Raising hands forward and up

- **Inhale** and raise your arms forward and up as you lower your left foot down to the floor.
- **Exhale** and, as your belly draws in and up, lower your arms and lift your right foot away from the floor.
- **Inhale** and lower your right foot back down.
- Repeat a few more times as if there was a piece of string from your navel to your knee and, as you **exhale**, your belly draws back and up which helps to lift your knee.

Warrior I with knee lifts

- Continue using your core to help you to balance. Start with your feet hip-distance apart and then step your left foot back. Can you be on the ball of the back foot with the back heel lifted? If that feels too much, lower your heel down and turn your left toes slightly out.
- **Inhale**, bend your right knee and raise your arms forward and up. Check your knee doesn't go beyond your ankle (see Figure 182).
- **Exhale** and push off from your left foot; step forward and lift your knee. See if you can balance on your right foot and keep your left foot hovering. You might find you can lift the knee high, or you may need to keep your toes close to the floor for more support (see Figure 181, page 261).
- **Inhale** and step gracefully back, raising your arms forward and up.
- Repeat.
- **Exhale** and put weight onto your front foot as you draw your belly in and up and lift your left knee up into the balance. Sense the lift of your leg coming from your belly.
- Repeat 3–4 more times.
- Then step forward to the front of your mat and pause. Notice what has happened to your breathing. Did it speed up? Are you aware of your heart beating? Of your lungs expanding? Can you come back into the moment just noticing the physical movement of breath in your body? Notice if you have thoughts or judgements about the pose or the balance or your body in the pose. Observe your thoughts and then come back to your breathing.
- Repeat on the other side.

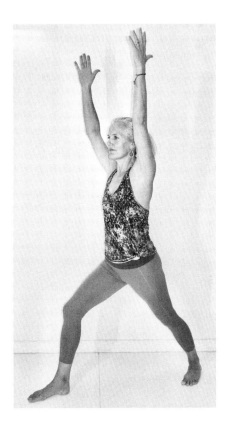

Figure 182: Warrior I with arms forward and up

Quad stretch

- You might want to be close to a wall for your balance.
- To stretch the muscles at the top of your thigh, draw your left knee in towards you. Slide your left hand down your shin and hold your ankle; then let your knee lengthen down to the floor as you take your leg behind you. You can hold onto a wall for support.
- Then bend your standing leg, draw your pubic bone towards your belly button so you tone your belly, soften your front ribs in and then start to straighten your standing leg.
- Lengthen your knee away from your hip so you get a stretch in your quadricep. Stay for a few breaths then change sides (see Figure 183).

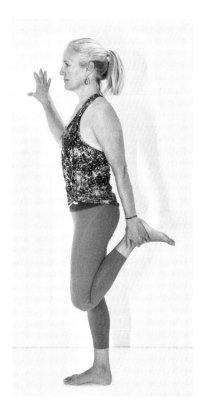

Figure 183: Standing quadricep stretch

- This same stretch can be done lying on your side or on your tummy if that is preferable to you. You can also use a strap to help you hold onto your foot.
- Repeat on the other side.

Hamstring stretch

- Lie on your back and bend both knees.
- Find the natural curves of your spine. Feel your rib cage and pelvis making contact with the mat or floor. Feel the space at your neck. Feel the space at your lower back.
- If you are not sure if your pelvis is neutral, **inhale** and arch your lower back and send your pubic bones away from you. **Exhale**, flatten your lower back and draw your pubic bones towards you. Then find somewhere in the middle.
- Draw your right knee in without changing the shape of your lower back.
- Place a strap or scarf around the ball of the foot, where it meets your arch. Then cross the strap in front of your leg and hold onto it, one end in each hand.
- Extend your foot in the strap towards the ceiling.
- Keep your spine neutral and use the strap to draw your thighbone down into your pelvis (see Figure 23, page 57).
- You can keep your left knee bent or, if it doesn't aggravate your lower back, you can straighten your leg out along the mat or floor. Press your left foot into an imaginary wall or you can even position yourself so that your foot can press into the wall. If this does cause any discomfort in your lower back, then re-bend your left knee and place the foot back onto the floor.
- Stay here for about 1 minute, breathing and feeling your breath move into your upper back, middle back and down into your lower back. Exhale out from your belly.
- To come out of this pose, bend both knees. Bring your feet back down to the mat/floor. Pause to observe the differences between your right and left legs. I also find if I straighten out my legs, my right leg now feels much longer than my left leg. You can explore if you feel the same.
- Repeat on the left side.

Daily strengthening exercises

Try to incorporate these strengthening moves into your daily life, even when you are fatigued.

- Every time you go to **sit down**, don't. Just before your bottom touches the seat stand back up. If you did this every time you went to sit down, including going to the toilet, you would be building strength without feeling like you were doing lots of repetitions of the chair pose. How many could you do in a day?
- When you **brush your teeth**, stand on one leg for the first minute and then stand on your opposite leg for the second minute.
- Core climbing: when you climb your stairs can you incorporate your core? **Exhale** and tone your belly as you lift your foot up onto each step.

Zzzzz – sleep and insomnia

We can be tired and wired. Physically our bodies are tired but when we lie down our mind becomes really active and busy with thoughts, and we can't sleep.

Breathing techniques

Alternate nostril breathing

Alternate nostril breathing is a wonderful breathing practice that helps to calm our overactive mind. One of our nostrils is always more dominant than the other and if you exhale out you might notice that one is more open than the other. This changes every 90 minutes or so and there is a moment when there is a balance between the two. According to yogic texts, our energy moves through our body via thousands of **nadis** or energy channels. The main energy channel runs along the spinal column and is known as the **sushumna nadis** which ends at the base of the nose between the two nostrils.

There are two other energy channels that swirl and spiral around the main channel. One runs to the end of the left nostril known as **ida** and the other ends at the end of the right nostril known as **pingala**. The left nostril is said to be cooling and calming and the right nostril is warming and energising. The flow of energy through the two nostrils is rarely equal as described, but by directing our breath in our nostrils we can directly affect the energy of our body and this breathing practice or pranayama can be balancing, calming or energising.

Chandra bhedana

Known as 'moon piercing breath', **chandra bhedana** involves breathing in through the left nostril and out through the right nostril to calm the mind. If you feel your nose from the top, you will feel firstly bone and then there is a point as you move down your nose to the tip where bone changes to cartilage (see Figure 184). At this point you might feel a little indentation in the side of your nose. This is the best point at which to close the nostrils, rather than at the end of the nose where they can sometimes get a bit stuck and this can make breathing become stressful, which is the opposite of what we are trying to achieve.

- Traditionally, you would bring your index and middle finger either to the base of your thumb (see Figure 185) or to a point between your eyebrows. This leaves your ring finger and thumb free to close your nostrils. However, if this is not accessible or if it is uncomfortable, use whichever fingers are easiest to use for closing the nostrils.

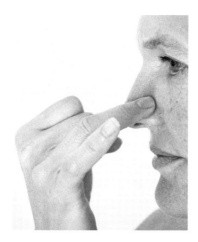

Figure 184: Feeling where to close the nostrils

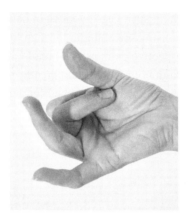

Figure 185: Using thumb and ring finger to close the left nostril

- Sit so that your spine is long, and on a support that allows you to keep the natural curves of your spine. As the yoga tradition sees energy as flowing along the spine, we don't want to restrict the movement of energy in the body by slumping or rounding the spine. Check that your head isn't dropping forward and start to watch your breathing as you breathe in and out.
- Then, closing off your right nostril, breathe out through your **left** and then **inhale** through the **left** and, at the top of your inhale, lightly close your **left** nostril and **breathe out** through your **right**.
- At the end of your exhale, lightly close your right nostril.
- **Breathe in** through your **left** nostril and, at the top of your **inhale**, close it.
- **Breathe out** through your **right** nostril.
- Continue breathing **in** through your **left** and **out** through your **right** for as long as you feel comfortable or until you start to feel that the steadying of your breath is beginning to have a more restful and peaceful effect on your mind.
- Check that your shoulders are relaxed as you hold your hand up to close your nostrils. If it becomes too much for that arm or if you are congested, lower your arm and instead visualise your breath going into your left nostril and out through the right. Visualise this alternate nostril breathing for a few rounds. You can even focus on your hands as you visualise the breath, opening up your left hand as you visualise breath moving in through your left nostril then closing your left hand and opening your right hand as you visualise breathing

269

out through your right nostril. Close your right hand and open up your left as you continue visualising breathing in through the left and out through the right, opening the respective palm as you breathe in or out through that side.

• Then breathe in through both nostrils and breathe out through both nostrils and see if you are ready to head back to bed for a good night's sleep.

Mudras and mantras

Chin and jnana mudra

You could also try using a hand gesture or mudra like **chin mudra** or **jnana mudra**. They are said to help clear our mind, which could be useful to help clear our head ready for sleep.

Bring the tip of your thumb to your index finger of the same hand and extend your other fingers. If you turn your palms to face up this is the jnana mudra or wisdom mudra; if you turn your palms to face down this is the chin mudra or consciousness mudra (see Figure 186).

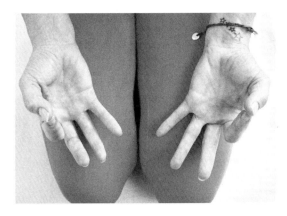

Figure 186: Palms up – the jnana mudra

I was always taught that you turn your palms up if you need to receive energy and turn your palms down if you want to conserve energy. The index finger is said to represent our individual consciousness and the thumb represents universal consciousness and by joining the two we connect ourselves to something bigger. According to *The Yoga Sutras of Patanjali*, if we can begin to calm the fluctuations of our mind, we start to glimpse our true nature or true self that is inherently calm and peaceful (sutra 1.3).[1]

So ham

If you find your mind is still buzzing and full of thoughts, try the **so ham** mantra (pronounced 'so hum') that mimics the sound of the breath to allow the mind to focus on something other than thoughts. So ham helps us to remember that we are all connected. and this connection can help us feel less isolated or lonely, especially at night.

Sleep

I find that when I can't sleep it helps to escape my bed and bedroom and move to another area to try to prepare for sleep so that my bed is somewhere that I, hopefully, come to sleep. However, you may prefer to sit up in bed or to do these practices lying down. If you want some gentle movement first, then you might want to follow the simple daily sequence (Figures 1 to 16, pages 19–29) in the 'Introduction', and as this sequence is done lying down it could also be done in your bed.

Coherent breathing

Our heart rate is measured in beats per minute. When we breathe in, our heart rate increases, and when we breathe out our heart rate decreases. Our hearts don't beat at a perfectly regular rhythm and the time between the beats is known as heart rate variability. Coherent breathing increases heart rate variability, which is good, as it means your heart rate is adjusting and is more flexible and responsive to changes in your breathing. A higher heart rate variability means our cardiovascular system is more flexible, more balanced and more resilient to stress.

In coherent breathing, we are working towards breathing at a rate of 5 breaths per minute, which generally translates into inhaling and exhaling to the count of '6'. However, this might be something that you need to build up to.

- Breathing in and out to counts helps you to stretch your breath but not strain it. So, start by taking a breath in and breathe out for 3, 2, 1.Then breathe in for 3, 2, 1.

- Then add a count. Breathe out 4, 3, 2, 1. Breathe in 4, 3, 2, 1. If this is challenging or you are finding it hard to breathe in and out for a count of 4, then go back to the count of 3.
- Now add a count. Breathe out 5, 4, 3, 2, 1. Breathe in 5, 4, 3, 2, 1.
- If counting in and out for 5 isn't straining your breath, then try adding a further count so that you breathe out 6, 5, 4, 3, 2, 1 and breathe in 6, 5, 4, 3, 2, 1. However, if you find that this is making you get out of breath or you are finding it hard to breathe in and out to this count, please come back to a count of 4 or 3.

You could also record yourself counting the inhale and the exhale and play this back to help you stay with the breathing. There are also various apps that use sound to help you stay with the count. The sounds can chime every 5 counts, or you can even adapt them to fit your breath count.

In *The Healing Power of the Breath*, Brown and Gerbarg describe how this technique shifts 'the stress-response system into a healthier balance by activating the healing, recharging part of the nervous system... the level of activity of this system can be measured using the natural fluctuations in heart rate that are linked to breathing; these fluctuations are used to calculate heart rate variability or HRV'.[2] HRV measures the balance between the sympathetic and parasympathetic nervous systems, remembering that our inhale stimulates the sympathetic side of the nervous system and makes our heart rate quicken and our exhale stimulates the soothing parasympathetic side of the nervous system, and makes our heart rate slow down. Ideally, we are working towards having a steady and smooth fluctuation in our heart rate. A good heart rate variability is a good measure of the balance between the two sides of the nervous system and, as a result, of our wellbeing.

Coherent breathing with supine twist

You could practise coherent breathing in a supine twist. This can help to keep your shoulders still and stop them moving up and down as you breathe in and out. If your shoulders stay resting on the mat, this allows you to bring your focus and breath down into your belly and feel the movement of your breath here instead of in your shoulders and neck.

- Lying on your back, stretch your arms out in line with your shoulders or find an angle that feels supportive.

- Take a breath in and, as you **exhale**, drop your knees over to one side. You can support your lower back by placing a cushion under your knees or between your thighs to keep your knees hip-distance apart (see Figure 21, page xx).
- Breathe for a few minutes, counting your breath. Then next time you exhale, let go of your breath and just observe how you feel.

Supported child's pose

This is another pose that can be very calming and help to draw your awareness inwards. Forward folds are energetically calming poses and, with the support of a bolster or blanket, you can start to feel your breath moving into the back of your body. Sense your clothing moving as your breath expands into body and sense your body soften as you exhale.

Taking your knees wide, toes touching, fold forward and place your forehead onto a bolster or some folded blankets. This is to help keep your spine, including your neck, long. If this is uncomfortable for your knees, you can create space at the back of your knees by placing a folded blanket on your calves so you rest your bottom on the blanket. If it feels uncomfortable at your hip creases, you can place a blanket on top of your thighs so you fold over the blanket and rest your tummy on the blanket, again creating space at the top of the thighs.(see Figure 36, page 73).

Yoga nidra

Yoga nidra or conscious deep 'yogic sleep' is an immensely powerful meditation technique that can be more effective than conventional sleep. It is said that 45 minutes of yogic sleep feels like three hours of conventional sleep but there isn't any scientific evidence to back this up. However, it definitely promotes deep rest and relaxation and teaches us how to relax on a deeper level.

Yoga nidra combines breath awareness, guided imagery and body sensing for the purpose of inducing a deep sense of peace. It is practised lying in the savasana pose, although it can be done seated and it can be done by anyone.

Start the nidra by setting an intention for the practice. Sense your body and breathing to help trigger the parasympathetic side of your nervous system and your relaxation response.

Research shows that measurement of brain activity (using electroencephalography – EEG) indicates that during yoga nidra participants are in a deeply relaxed state similar to that of sleep. The brain shifts from beta, the awakened state with lots of brain activity, to alpha the more relaxed state. In alpha, serotonin is released which is believed to help boost your mood and aid sleep. From alpha we shift into deep alpha and high theta brain-wave state where our thoughts slow down to four to eight per second. In theta we can have random thoughts, see images, colours and visions, or even hear the voice of someone talking.

From theta we can be guided into delta, which is the most restorative state. Stress in our lives can mean that lots of people do not go into deep states of sleep like theta and delta on a regular basis. This form of meditation can help cells regenerate and repair and to decrease anxiety, lower blood pressure and improve mood.

So that you can experience yoga nidra you can access a 20-minute recorded yoga nidra on my website: www.vickyfox-yoga.com.

Finding time, developing a practice

Now that you have read through the various yoga practices in this book you can start to fit them into your life. Put into practice what you have read, find out what really resonates with you and build your own toolbox of poses and sequences that ease your side effects, calm your mind or give you a sense of being whole. If it feels a little daunting then start small. Be honest with how much time you think you can dedicate to your wellbeing, and start with that. Regularity is the key to building a habit so find a few things that you feel are going to benefit you the most and observe what happens if you dedicate some time every day to those.

Is there a good time of day for you to practise? If you share your home with other people, maybe let them know that you are taking some time out for yourself and that you might need some encouragement or some space from family members that is your 'me time'. If you have small children or pets, you might just have to incorporate them into your practice, letting them explore some of the movements with you. Children are curious by nature and may enjoy following you through some yoga poses or breathing techniques.

Create some space by turning off your computer or putting your phone on silent and, if you have a mat, roll it out to signify the start of your precious yoga time. You might have your yoga props or a certain cushion that you always sit on when you do yoga; again, these just mark the beginning of your practice. You might even light a candle, have uplifting photos or pictures, or place some flowers in the room to create a more sacred special space for your practice.

Remember that yoga is not just physical poses that have to be done on a yoga mat. Yoga includes breathing, mantras, meditation, mudras and, most importantly, ways to rest and relax which are so important when helping our bodies to repair. So you may not even have a dedicated time or place at home where you practise. You might use breathing techniques whilst travelling, having chemotherapy, or waiting for appointments. We spend a lot of time waiting and sometimes it is that being in limbo that can be incredibly stressful so explore if one of the breathing techniques helps reduce your feelings of stress or anxiety. Was there something that gave you a break and allowed your body to still and your mind to quieten? A body scan or just some quiet time with your eyes closed exploring sensations in your body?

Stick some reminders around your house that help you do some small things often. Post some reminders to 'breathe' around your house; stick them to your mirror, your fridge or your doors. Add daily reminders to your phone to 'Pause and breathe'. Notice your posture every time you sit and, if it helps, put a reminder on your computer screen to have a 'long neutral spine'. Maybe your notes will remind you to repeat a mantra or positive affirmation. You can do some of the seated poses whilst sitting at your desk or you can practise some of the eye exercises when you have been on your computer for a long time and add other standing poses to other spaces in your day.

I hope you enjoy the practices in this book and that they can support you in the same way they have helped students in my classes. Now it is over to you. This book is just your guide and you are the best teacher. You know what it feels like to be in your body and you are the only one who can put aside time for *you*. You have the power to put yourself and your wellbeing first. This book can give you the foundations to grow, to establish deep roots that keep you grounded and strong when life is blowing you off centre, and with those strong roots you can embrace a sense of gratitude to yourself. This is definitely a great starting point, being thankful to yourself for opening this book and exploring how yoga might benefit your side effects. And if you do put it into practice and that practice grows, then this is only the beginning of your yoga journey. Yoga might just hook you like it did me and you will constantly be learning, growing, and evolving instead of revolving.

https://vickyfox-yoga.com/yoga-for-cancer-classes
@yogaforcancer

References

Introduction

1. Macmillan Cancer Support. *Physical Activity for People with Metastatic Bone Disease*. 2021. Available at: www.macmillan.org.uk/healthcare-professionals/news-and-resources/guides/physical-activity-for-people-with-metastatic-bone-disease (Accessed: 12 January 2022).
2. Hendersen E. Many cancer survivors continue to suffer long-term burdensome symptoms, study shows. *News-Medical.Net*, 20 September 2021. Available at: www.news-medical.net/news/20210920/Many-cancer-survivors-continue-to-suffer-long-term-burdensome-symptoms-study-shows.aspx (Accessed: 11 January 2022).
3. Cancer Research UK *Exercise Guidelines for Cancer Patients*. 2019. Available at: www.cancerresearchuk.org/about-cancer/coping/physically/exercise-guidelines (Accessed: 8 February 2022).
4. National Cancer Institute (NIH). *Physical Activity and Cancer*. 2020. Available at: www.cancer.gov/about-cancer/causes-prevention/risk/obesity/physical-activity-fact-sheet (Accessed: 11 January 2022).
5. Garritt C. *Get Your Oomph Back: a guide to exercise after a cancer diagnosis* London, UK: Hammersmith Health Books; 2021.

How to use this book

1. Satchidananda SS (Translator). *The Yoga Sutras of Patanjali*. New edn.

Buckingham, VA, USA: Integral Yoga International; 2012.

2. Kabat-Zinn J. *Full Catastrophe Living: how to cope with stress, pain and illness using mindfulness meditation*. Revised edn. London, UK: Piatkus; 2013.

3. Spiegel D, Bloom JR, Kraemer HC, Gottheil E. Effects of psychosocial treatment on survival of patients with metastatic breast cancer. *The Lancet* 1989; 2(8668): 888–891.

4. Fawzy F, Fawzy N, Hyun C, Elashoff R, Guthrie D, Fahey J, Morton D. Malignant melanoma; effects of an early structured psychiatric intervention, coping, and affective state on recurrence and survival six years later. *Archives of General Psychiatry* 1993; 50(9): 681–689.

5. Reynolds P, Boyd PT, Blacklow RS, Jackson JS, Greenberg RS, Austin DF, Chen VW, Edwards BK. The relationship between social ties and survival among black and white breast cancer patients: National Cancer Institute black/white survival study group cancer epidemiology, biomarkers, and prevention. *Cancer Epidemiol Biomarkers Prev* 1994; 3(3): 253–259.

6. Penninx BW, van Tilburg TG, Kriegsman DMW, Deeg DJH. Effects of social support and personal coping resources on mortality in older age; the longitudinal aging study Amsterdam. *American Journal of Epidemiology* 1997; 146(6): 510–590.

7. Giles L, Glonek G, Luszcz M, Andrews G. Effect of social networks on 10 year survival in very old Australians; the Australian longitudinal study of aging. *Journal of Epidemiology and Community Health* 2005; 59(7): 574–579.

8. Banerjee B, Vadiraj HS, Ram A, Rao R, Jaypal M, Gopinath KS, Ramesh BS, Rao N, Kumar A, Raghuram N, Hegde S, Nagendra HR, Hande MP. Effects of an integrated yoga program in modulating psychological stress and radiation-induced genotoxic stress in breast cancer patients undergoing radiotherapy. *Integrative Cancer Therapies* 2007; 6(3): 242–250.

9. Sovik R. A mantra meditation for everyone. *Yoga International* 2022. Available at: https://yogainternational.com/article/view/a-mantra-meditation-for-everyone (Accessed 9 February 2022).

Anxiety

1. Sovik R. *Moving Inward: the journey to meditation*. Honesdale, PA: Himalayan Institute Press; 2006.

2. Gilbert P. *The Compassionate Mind: compassion focused therapy*. London: Constable; 2010.
3. Hanson R. *Buddha's Brain: the practical neuroscience of happiness, love and wisdom*. Oakland, CA: New Harbinger; 2009.
4. Satchidananda SS (Translator). *The Yoga Sutras of Patanjali*. New edn. Buckingham, VA, USA: Integral Yoga International; 2012.

Breathing

1. . Rama S, Ballentine R, Hymes A. *Science of Breath: a practical guide*. Honesdale, PA: Himalayan Institute Press; 1999.
2. Desikachar TKV. *The Heart of Yoga: developing a personal practice*. Rochester, VT, USA: Inner Traditions; 1995.
3. Nestor J. *Breath: the new science of a lost art*. London, UK: Penguin; 2021.

Chemo brain

1. Macmillan Cancer Support. *Cognitive Changes: chemo brain*. 2018. Available at: www.macmillan.org.uk/cancer-information-and-support/impacts-of-cancer/chemo-brain (Accessed: 11 January 2022).
2. Lim S-A, Cheong K-J. Regular yoga practice improves antioxidant status, immune function, and stress hormone releases in young healthy people: a randomized, double-blind, controlled pilot study. *J Alternative Complementary Medicine* 2015; 21(9): 530–538. Available at: www.ncbi.nlm.nih.gov/pubmed/26181573 (Accessed: 11 January 2022).
3. Ashcraft KA, Warner AB, Jones LW, Dewhirst DVM. Exercise as adjunct therapy in cancer. *Seminars in Radiation Oncology* 2019; 29(1): 16–24.
4. Hirschi G. *Mudras – yoga in your hands*. London, UK: Coronet; 2016.
5. Alzheimer Research and Prevention Foundation *Practice the 12-minute yoga meditation exercise*. 2022. Available at: https://alzheimersprevention.org/research/kirtan-kriya-yoga-exercise/ (Accessed: 11 January 2022).

Colostomy, ostomy, ileostomy and yoga with a stoma

1. Russell S. *The Bowel Cancer Recovery Toolkit*. London, UK: Hammersmith Health Books; 2020.
2. Howard L. *Pelvic Liberation: using yoga, self-inquiry and breath awareness for pelvic health*. Emeryville, CA: Leslie Howard Yoga; 2017.

Cramps

1. Howard L. *Pelvic Liberation: using yoga, self-inquiry and breath awareness for pelvic health*. Emeryville, CA: Leslie Howard Yoga; 2017.

Fatigue

1. Hendersen E. Many cancer survivors continue to suffer long-term burdensome symptoms, study shows. *News-Medical.Net* 20 September 2021. Available at: www.news-medical.net/news/20210920/Many-cancer-survivors-continue-to-suffer-long-term-burdensome-symptoms-study-shows.aspx (Accessed: 11 January 2022).
2. Kiecolt-Glaser JK, Bennett JM, Andridge R, Peng J, et al. Yoga's impact on inflammation, mood, and fatigue in breast cancer survivors: a randomized controlled trial. *Journal of Clinical Oncology* 2014; 32(10). Available at: https://ascopubs.org/doi/full/10.1200/JCO.2013.51.8860 (Accessed: 11 January 2022).
3. Hirschi G. *Mudras – yoga in your hands*. London, UK: Coronet; 2016.

Grief

1. Macmillan Cancer Support (2021) *Contact us*. Available at: www.macmillan.org.uk/about-us/contact-us (Accessed: 12 January 2022).

Hot flushes

1. Lasater JH. *Relax and renew: restful yoga for stressful times*. Boulder, CO, US: Rodmell Press; 2011.

Immune system and infections

1. Cohen S. If you want to boost immunity, look to the gut. *UCLA Health* 19 March 2021. Available at: https://connect.uclahealth.org/2021/03/19/want-to-boost-immunity-look-to-the-gut/ (Accessed: 8 February 2022).
2. Lotter E. Your gut is the cornerstone of your immune system. *Health24* 18 March 2016. Available at: www.news24.com/health24/medical/flu/preventing-flu/your-gut-is-the-cornerstone-of-your-immune-system-20160318 (Accessed: 8 February 2022).
3. Furness JB, Kunze WAA, Clerc N. II. The intestine as a sensory organ: neural, endocrine, and immune responses. *American Journal of Physiology – Gastrointestinal and Liver Physiology* 1999; 277(5): G922-G928. Available at: https://journals.physiology.org/doi/full/10.1152/ajpgi.1999.277.5.g922 (Accessed: 8 February 2022)
4. Lumen. *Cortisol and immunity*. Available at: https://courses.lumenlearning.com/boundless-ap/chapter/stress-and-immunity/ (Accessed: 12 January 2022).
5. McClelland DC, Kirshnit C. The effect of motivational arousal through films on salivary immunoglobulin A. *Psychology and Health* 1988; 2(1): 31–52.
6. Raisingchildren.net.au (2019) *Touch, holding and massage for your premature baby in the NICU*. Available at: https://raisingchildren.net.au/newborns/premature-babies/connecting-communicating/touch-massage-in-the-nicu (Accessed: 8 February 2022).
7. Harding K. *The rabbit effect: live longer, happier, and healthier with the groundbreaking science of kindness*. New York: Atria Books; 2019.
8. Hamilton D. *The Five Side Effects of Kindness: this book will make you feel better, be happier and live longer*. London: Hay House UK; 2017.
9. Lerman B, Harricharran T, Ogunwobi OO. Oxytocin and cancer: an emerging link. *World Journal of Clinical Oncology* 2018; 9(5): 74–82.
10. Steptoe A, Dockray S, Wardle J. Positive effect and psychobiological processes

relevant to health', *Journal of Personality* 2009; 77(6): 1747–1776.

11. Szeto A, Nation DA, Mendez AJ, Dominguez-Bendala J, et al. Oxytocin attenuates NADPH dependent superoxide activity and il-6 secretion in macrophages and vascular cells. *American Journal of Physiology: Endocrinology and Metabolism* 2008; 295(6): E1495–E1501.

12. Kiecolt-Glaser JK, Bennett JM, Andridge R, Peng J, et al. Yoga's impact on inflammation, mood, and fatigue in breast cancer survivors: a randomized controlled trial. *Journal of Clinical Oncology* 2014; 32(10): . Available at: https://ascopubs.org/doi/full/10.1200/JCO.2013.51.8860 (Accessed: 11 January 2022).

13. Fredrickson B, Cohn MA, Coffey KA, Pek J, Finkel SM. Open hearts build lives: positive emotions, induced through loving kindness meditation build consequential personal resources. *Journal of Personality and Social Psychology*, 2008; 95(5): 1045–1062.

14. Sri Swami Satchidananda (Translator) *The yoga sutras of Patanjali*. New edn. Buckingham, VA, USA: Integral Yoga International; 2012.

15. Dunn L. Be thankful: science says gratitude is good for your health. *Today* 26 November 2015. Available at: www.today.com/health/be-thankful-science-says-gratitude-good-your-health-t58256 (Accessed: 12 January 2022).

16. Ruini C, Vescovelli F. The role of gratitude in breast cancer: its relationship with post traumatic growth, psychological well-being and distress. *Journal of Happiness Studies* 2012; 14(1): 263-274. Available at: www.researchgate.net/publication/257589163_The_Role_of_Gratitude_in_Breast_Cancer_Its_Relationships_with_Post-traumatic_Growth_Psychological_Well-Being_and_Distress (Accessed: 8 February 2022).

17. Wood AM, Joseph S, Lloyd J, Atkins S. Gratitude influences sleep through the mechanism of pre-sleep cognitions. *Journal of Psychosomatic Research* 2009; 66(1): 43–48.

18. Kornfield J. *Buddha's Little Instruction Book*. London: Rider Books; 1996.

19. Turner KA. *Radical Remission: surviving cancer against all odds*. London: Bravo Ltd; 2014.

Lymphoedema

1. Cancer Research UK (2019) *Lowering your risk of lymphoedema*. Available at: www.cancerresearchuk.org/about-cancer/coping/physically/lymphoedema-and-

cancer/lowering-your-risk (Accessed: 8 February 2022).

2. Lane K, Worsley D, Mckenzie D. Exercise and the lymphatic system: implications for breast-cancer survivors. *Sports Medicine* 2005; 35(6): 461–471.

3. Steinberg L. *Iyengar yoga cancer book*. 2013. Available at: www.loissteinberg. com/products/iyengar-yoga-cancer-book-2013 (Accessed: 12 January 2022).

4. Lymphoedema Support Network (LSN) (2021) *About cellulitis*. Available at: www.lymphoedema.org/cellulitis/about-cellulitis/ (Accessed: 12 January 2022).

Menopause

1. Howard L. *Pelvic liberation: using yoga, self-inquiry and breath awareness for pelvic health*. Emeryville, CA: Leslie Howard Yoga; 2017.

2. Lasater JH. *Relax and Renew: restful yoga for stressful times*. Boulder, CO: Rodmell Press; 2011.

Nausea

1. Hirschi G. *Mudras – yoga in your hands*. London: Coronet; 2016.

Osteoporosis

1. Meng-Xia Ji, Qi Yu. Primary osteoporosis in menopausal women. *Chronic Dis Transl Med* 2015; 1(1): 9–13. Available at: www.ncbi.nlm.nih.gov/pmc/articles/PMC5643776/ (Accessed: 12 January 2022).

2. NHS *Osteosporosis*. 2019. Available at: www.nhs.uk/conditions/osteoporosis/ (Accessed: 12 January 2022).

3. Fishman LM, Saltonstall E. Yoga for osteoporosis: a pilot study. *Topics in Geriatric Rehabilitation* 2009; 25(3): 244-250. Available at: https://journals. lww.com/topicsingeriatricrehabilitation/Fulltext/2009/07000/Yoga_for_ Osteoporosis__A_Pilot_Study.9.aspx (Accessed: 12 January 2022).

Peripheral neuropathy

1. Keller D. *Yoga as therapy fundamentals* [unpublished course workbook]. Additional credit for fascia flossing exercises to Zephyr Wildman: Zephyr Yoga Online. 2014. Available at: https://zephyryoga.com/ (Accessed: 8 February 2022).

Referred pain

1. International Association for the Study of Pain (IASP) (2017) *Terminology.* Available at: www.iasp-pain.org/resources/terminology/#pain (Accessed: 12 January 2022).
2. Peppone L, Janelsins MC, Kamen C, Mohile SG, et al. (2015) The effect of YOCAS yoga for musculoskeletal symptoms among breast cancer survivors on hormonal therapy. *Breast Cancer Research and Treatment* 2015; 150: 597-604.
3. Ross A, Thomas SA. (2010) The health benefits of yoga and exercise: a review of comparison studies. *Journal of Alternative and Complementary Medicine* 2010; 16(1): 3-12.
4. Hassan J, Courtoise I, Van den Bergh O, Vlaeyen JWS, Van Diest I. Pain and respiration a systematic review. *Pain* 2017; 158(6): 995–1006. Available at: https://pubmed.ncbi.nlm.nih.gov/28240995/ (Accessed: 12 January 2022).
5. Ornish D. *Love and Survival: the scientific basis for the healing power of intimacy.* New York: William Morrow; 1999.
6. Donaldson M. Resilient to pain: a model of how yoga may decrease interference among people experiencing chronic pain. *Explore (NY)* 2019; 15(3): 230–238. Available at: www.ncbi.nlm.nih.gov/pmc/articles/PMC6517077/ (Accessed: 12 January 2022).
7. Burch V, Penman D. *Mindfulness for Health: a practical guide to relieving pain, reducing stress and restoring wellbeing.* London: Piatkus; 2013.

Scar tissue

1. Muktibohananda S. *Hatha Yoga Pradipika.* Fort Munger, Bihar, India: Bihar School of Yoga; 1998.

Weakness in muscles – building strength

1. Volpi E, Nazemi R, Fujita S. Muscle tissue changes with aging. *Curr Opin Clin Nutr Metab Care* 2004; 7(4): 405-410. www.ncbi.nlm.nih.gov/labs/pmc/articles/PMC2804956/
2. J Lewis. The impacts of inactivity. The Osteoperformance Clinic; 2017. www.osteoperformance.co.uk/blogs/the-impacts-of-inactivity/
3. Jiricka MK. Activity tolerance and fatigue pathophysiology: concepts of altered health states. In: Porth CM (ed). *Essentials of Pathophysiology: Concepts of Altered Health States*. Philadelphia, PA: Lippincott Williams & Wilkins; 2008.
4. Having more muscle mass may mean milder chemotherapy side effects. breastcancer.org 3 March 2017. www.breastcancer.org/research-news/more-muscle-mass-may-mean-less-chemo-sfx
5. Macmillan Cancer Support. *Physical activity for people with metastatic bone disease*. 2021. Available at: www.macmillan.org.uk/healthcare-professionals/news-and-resources/guides/physical-activity-for-people-with-metastatic-bone-disease (Accessed: 12 January 2022).

Zzzz – sleep and insomnia

1. Sri Swami Satchidananda (Translator) *The yoga sutras of Patanjali*. New edn. Buckingham, VA, USA: Integral Yoga International; 2012.
2. Brown RP, Gerbarg P. *The healing power of the breath: simple techniques to reduce stress and anxiety, enhance concentration, and balance your emotions*. Boston, MA: Shambhala; 2012.

Glossary of yoga terms

Agni: Digestive fire.

Ahimsa: Ahimsa is the first of the 'eight limbs' of yoga and means non-harming or non-violence. Non-harming in the way we treat others and ourselves. Ahimsa is not just the absence of violence, but it is the presence of love.

Anandamaya kosha: Fifth layer or sheath of the koshas, the bliss body.

Annamaya kosha: First layer or sheath of the koshas, the physical or gross body.

Anuloma viloma: This is also known as alternate nostril breathing and can also be balancing and calming.

Apana vaya mudra: A mudra focusing on downward-moving energy formed by bringing your index fingers to the base of your thumb and then bringing your ring and middle finger to the tip of the thumb. Apana is one of the prana vayas that focuses on elimination.

Apanasana: Wind-relieving pose.

Asana: Posture or seat. According to Patanjali, asana is a steady and comfortable meditative pose or seat.

Bija: One-syllable mantras that have a particular vibration.

Chandra bhedana: Known as 'moon piercing breath'; 'chandra' meaning moon and 'bhedana' meaning piercing or entering. It involves breathing in through the left nostril and breathing out through the right nostril to calm the mind. Activates the ida nadi and is calming and cooling.

Chin mudra: Bring the tip of the thumb to your index finger and extend your other fingers. If you then turn your palms to face down this is chin mudra or consciousness mudra.

Gayatri mantra: A mantra for gratitude which gives thanks to the sun that is forever giving and never receiving, with the wish that the sun might shine through and inspire all of us.

Hakini mudra: Bringing the fingertips of each hand together like a tee pee or tent; said to be a mudra for the mind.

Ham: A one-syllable mantra relating to help cleanse or balance energy at the throat.

Ida nadi: Major energy channel that runs along the spine to the end of the left nostril and is said to be cooling and calming.

Jnana mudra: Bring the tip of the thumb to your index finger and extend your other fingers. If you then turn your palms to face up this is jnana mudra or wisdom mudra.

Joint mudra: The right-hand thumb to ring finger and left-hand thumb to middle finger is said to balance energy into the joints.

Koshas: The yoga tradition of viewing the body as multi-layered sheaths or bodies that are all linked.

Lam: A one-syllable mantra relating to the base of the spine helping to clear stuck energy in this area and to give a sense of grounding or being more connected to the earth.

Manomaya kosha: Our mental sheath or body where we process our experiences.

Mantras: Sacred sounds that can be used as tools for meditation. 'Man' means 'mind' and 'tra' means 'to protect from', so these mantras help protect our mind. 'Tra' can also be translated as 'tool' so 'mantra' can also mean a tool for the mind.

Metta meditation: From Pali, meaning positive energy and kindness, this is a Buddhist meditation designed to create loving kindness for all beings, including ourselves.

Mudras: Literally meaning 'gesture', this term can refer to a hand position, eye position or even asanas or breathing techniques.

Mukula mudra: Beak mudra for healing; bring the fingers of one hand to touch your thumb and repeat the same with the opposite hand.

Nadis: A complex, subtle system of energy channels which flow through the body nourishing our muscles, organs and cells.

Om: A one-syllable mantra relating to the roof of the mouth and the point between the eyebrows. Yoga tradition describes it as the cosmic vibration of the universe.

Pingala nadi: An energy channel that runs along the spine to the end of the right nostril and is said to be warming or energising.

Prana: The vital energy or life force that flows through the body, sustaining life and creation. We can influence the flow of prana through breathing techniques.

Prana mudra: A mudra to help encourage the prana or energy into the body. Bring the thumb, little and ring finger to touch on both hands.

Pranamayakosha: Subtle layer of the body of breath or energy.

Pranayama: 'Ayama' means to stretch or extend and 'prana' is the energy that keeps us alive. Simon Low also taught me that 'pra' means consistent, 'prana' means life force and 'ayama' means to stretch, so that pranayama is a consistent practice of breathing techniques that help the flow of prana.

Prithivi mudra: A bone-strengthening mudra bringing the thumb and ring fingers to touch on both hands.

Pushan mudra: A mudra helpful for nausea and flatulence: on the right-hand, the tips of thumb, index and middle finger are touching. On the left-hand, the tips of the thumb, middle and ring finger are touching.

Ram: A one-syllable mantra relating to the abdomen and lower back helping to clear and balance energy in the navel centre.

Santosha: Contentment, being comfortable or okay with the way things are. One of the niyamas of *Patanjali's Yoga Sutras* (2.42).

Sat nam: A mantra meaning 'my true essence' or 'I am truth'; also, a bija mantra.

Savasana: Final resting pose where you are relaxed but conscious. All the doing is done, and you can be a human being.

Sitali/sikali: Cooling breathing techniques.

So ham: A mantra meaning 'I am that', 'I am connected to everyone and everything'. It reminds us of our interconnectedness.

Supta baddha konasana: A restorative pose to open up the belly and groin area. 'Supta' means 'lying supine', 'baddha' means 'bound' and 'kona' means 'angle'.

Surya bhedana pranayama: Alternative nostril breathing for stimulus and energy. 'Surya' means the Sun and 'bhedana' means piercing or entering. A more heating or energising practice activates pingala nadi.

Sushumna nadis: The main energy channel running along the spinal column from the base of the spine to the top of the nostrils.

Sutras: 'Sutras' mean 'threads', or short pieces of text threaded together.

Tadasana: The mountain pose, a grounded standing posture that helps to create a healthy alignment that you can keep throughout all the other poses or asanas.

Tapas: One of the niyamas, meaning practice. It refers to keeping the body cleansed by aligning our postures, habits, breathing, work and relaxation.

Trikonasana: The triangle pose, an energising pose that stretches upper and lower body and strengthens core muscles.

Vam: A one-syllable mantra cleansing and balancing energy in the lower belly and abdomen.

Vijnyanamaya kosha: Our intuitive or wisdom sheath or layer of the body.

Viloma 1: 'Vi' means 'against' and 'loma' means 'hair', so 'viloma' means against the natural flow and is a breathing technique for controlling the breath. It can be used to energise the body if it focuses on inhale. (Viloma 2 focuses on exhale.)

Vinyasa yoga: 'Nyasa' means 'to place' and 'vi' means in a 'special way'. Vinyasa yoga is a series of asanas that are sequenced in a special way to have certain desired effects. A gradual progression moving with breath to achieve union of breath and movement.

Viparita karani: 'Legs up the wall'; a pose which is calming for the nervous system. 'Viparita' means 'inverted' and 'karani' means 'in action'. The pose helps by turning the body upside down to give it a break from its normal functioning of having to pump blood back towards the heart

Virasana: This is the Hero's pose, a stable, seated pose for meditation or breathing practices.

Vishnu (or mrigi) mudra: This is a mudra where the index and middle finger are placed on the base of the thumb, leaving the ring finger and the thumb to close off the nostrils. It is often used in alternate nostril breathing.

Yam: A one-syllable mantra balancing energy around the heart, lungs and thoracic spine.

Yoga: A state of union between body and mind, individual and universal awareness.

Yoga nidra: 'Yoga sleep'. An immensely powerful meditation technique that can be more effective than conventional sleep, where the conscious mind is asleep, but awareness remains active.

Yoni mudra: A mudra or hand gesture which helps with menopausal symptoms – thumbs together, fingers pointing down.

Index

*Footnote: Bold page numbers refer to the glossary. Figures are comprehensively referred to from the text. Therefore, significant items in figures have only been given a page reference in the absence of their concomitant mention in the text referring to that figure.

*Footnote: Bold page numbers refer to the glossary. Figures are comprehensively referred to from the text. Therefore, significant items in figures have only been given a page reference in the absence of their concomitant mention in the text referring to that figure.

*Footnote: Bold page numbers refer to the glossary. Figures are comprehensively referred to from the text. Therefore, significant items in figures have only been given a page reference in the absence of their concomitant mention in the text referring to that figure.

*Footnote: Bold page numbers refer to the glossary. Figures are comprehensively referred to from the text. Therefore, significant items in figures have only been given a page reference in the absence of their concomitant mention in the text referring to that figure.

*Footnote: Bold page numbers refer to the glossary. Figures are comprehensively referred to from the text. Therefore, significant items in figures have only been given a page reference in the absence of their concomitant mention in the text referring to that figure.